Foreword

When asking young doctors why they wish to embark on haematology as a specialty, a thoroughly rehearsed answer centres around their interest for a combination of clinical and laboratory work. This, of course, is precisely what has attracted many of us to haematology, and it has been a challenge to writers, editors and publishers. Haematology has received increasing attention in the medical curriculum, and at the moment it features prominently in medical bookshops and libraries. However, in most cases students or trainees find they must choose between a laboratory-oriented atlas or a clinically-oriented book, ranging from 'lecture notes' to the more ponderous tomes.

Dr Mehta has chosen to straddle the two components of the subject in an original way, by presenting his material in the form of examples from real life. He has capitalised on a wealth of experience accumulated over the years, both in the diagnostic laboratory and in the haematology wards and clinics of major teaching hospitals. The result is a richly illustrated book in which informative microphotographs predictably abound, as they are the lot of day-to-day haematological practice; but the reader will be pleasantly surprised to find also a variety of other equally informative iconography, including photographs of skin changes, histological sections, CT images, and of course the occasional Southern blot. Rare as well as common conditions are illustrated.

I believe the natural readership of this book will consist of trainees in general internal medicine or haematology, and advanced medical students; medical laboratory scientists and technologists will also find the book most useful. It is likely to be particularly coveted by candidates for specialty and sub-specialty board examinations in the USA, by candidates for membership exams of Royal Colleges in the UK, and by candidates for equivalent ordeals in any other country. Indeed, it is clear from the broad range of clinical problems tackled that Atul Mehta has had pathology from different parts of the world before his eyes. At the same time, he has constantly had in mind a basic tenet of education, that learning should be enjoyable. For more experienced haematologists, I think the temptation to test their own prowess will be irresistible. I cannot claim that I solved all the riddles, but perhaps I could still pass an exam: just as with cryptic crosswords, the great gratification for cramming is when you get it right! To supplement the quiz solutions, the answer sections are generously enriched with numerous notes on clinical features, diagnosis and treatment that will be of use beyond passing exams.

I can only take pride in my past association with Dr Atul Mehta over several years, and it is my pleasure to wish this book the success it richly deserves.

Lucio Luzzatto, MD
Chairman, Department of Human Genetics
Attending Physician in Hematology
Memorial Sloan-Kettering Cancer Center
New York, NY, USA*

* *Formerly* Professor of Haematology, Royal Postgraduate Medical School, and Consultant Haematologist, Hammersmith Hospital, London, UK: Director, International Institute of Genetics and Biophysics, Napoli, Italy; Professor of Haematology and Consultant Haematologist, University College Hospital, Ibadan, Nigeria.

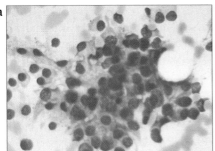

1a

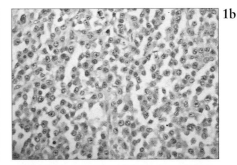

1b

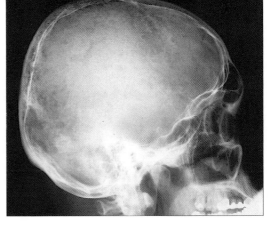

1c

1 A 76-year-old man has a 2-week history of abdominal pain, polyuria and nocturia. He has also noticed a skin nodule which is increasing in size. Investigations show:

Hb	7.1 g/dl
WBC	4.6 x 10⁹/l
Platelets	112 x 10⁹/l
Urea	46 mmol/l
Creatinine	905 mmol/l
Ca^{2+}	3.60 mmol/l (N 2.1–2.6 mmol/l)
Albumin	26 g/l (N 35–42 g/l)
Total protein	120 g/l (N 65–80 g/l)
Alkaline phosphatase	143 U/l (N 30–130 U/l)
Uric acid	0.48 mmol/l (N 0.3–0.4 mmol/l)

i. Comment on the above results.
ii. Comment on the bone marrow aspirate (1a).
iii. Comment on the aspirate of this patient's skin nodule (1b).
iv. Comment on the skull X-ray (1c).
v. What is the diagnosis?
vi. How should he be treated?

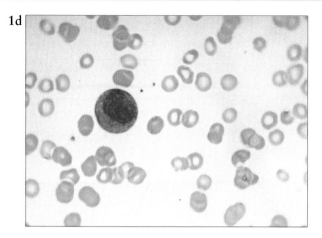

1d

1 i. The results indicate anaemia and thrombocytopenia with marked renal failure. Hypercalcaemia with normal alkaline phosphatase suggests primary bone marrow malignancy. The raised total protein suggests myeloma.

ii. The bone marrow is infiltrated by plasma cells, confirming myeloma. Plasma cell leukaemia is an aggressive form of myeloma characterised by large numbers of circulating plasma cells (**1d**).

iii. The skin deposit is also due to myeloma infiltration.

iv. The skull X-ray shows multiple lytic lesions, a characteristic finding in myeloma.

v. Myeloma.

vi. The hypercalcaemia and renal failure require urgent therapy with rehydration to promote diuresis. An IVU should not be done as the patient should not be dehydrated. However, abdominal ultrasound scan to exclude renal obstruction is valuable in acute renal failure.

Once baseline tests (paraprotein quantification in serum and urine, skeletal survey, beta-2 microglobulin and C Reactive Protein) are done, the patient should receive allopurinol (at a reduced dose of 100 mg/day because of his renal failure) followed by steroid therapy for hypercalcaemia. If the calcium remains elevated, consider biphosphonates, eg, pamidronate, given by slow intravenous infusion (15–60 mg, as a divided dose in renal failure). Chemotherapy should be commenced once he is stabilised. Cyclophosphamide (with steroids) is preferred in renal failure, as it is metabolised by the liver. Once his renal failure is improved, he could continue chemotherapy, either with melphalan and (intermittent oral) prednisolone, or with combination chemotherapy (eg, adriamycin, BCNU, cyclophosphamide, and melphalan – ABCM; or vincristine, adriamycin, both by infusion, and dexamethasone – VAD).

Interferon therapy may improve the response to chemotherapy and prolong duration of the stable ('plateau') phase of the disease that is often achieved after 4–6 cycles of chemotherapy. Long-term biphosphonate therapy (eg, sodium clodronate) may slow progress of skeletal disease in myeloma.

Younger patients (those under 65) with myeloma may benefit from intensive therapy, including autologous transplant of postchemotherapy marrow or peripheral blood stem cells. Patients under 50 who have an HLA-matching sibling should be considered for allogeneic bone marrow transplantation.

2a
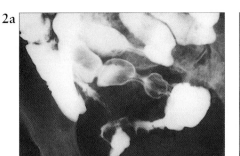

2b
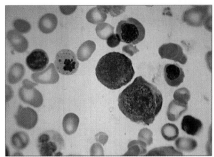

2c
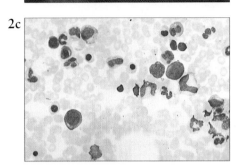

2d
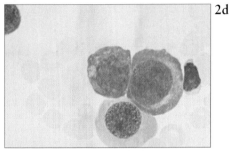

2 A 42-year-old woman gives a 2–3 month history of abdominal pain, diarrhoea and rectal bleeding. She passes blood-stained motions 4–6 times each day. She has also developed progressive tiredness and loss of appetite. On examination she is pale. There is no lymphadenopathy. She has mild generalised abdominal tenderness, but there is no organomegaly. A blood count shows:

Hb	8.4 g/dl
MCV	110 fl
WBC	3.1 x 10⁹/l
Platelets	80 x 10⁹/l

Biochemistry is normal, but the ESR is raised at 86 mm/hour.

i. What diagnosis is suggested by the barium meal and follow-through (2a)?
ii. What abnormalities are seen in her bone marrow aspirate (2b–2d)? What is the diagnosis?
iii. What further investigations would you perform?

2e

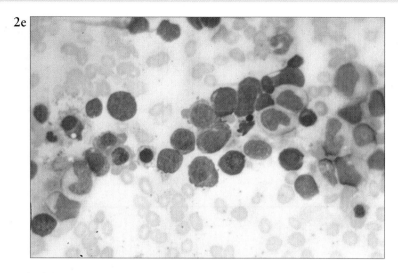

2 i. The barium meal and follow-through show classical changes of Crohn's disease. There is evidence of mucosal thickening and oedema with flocculation of barium.

ii. The bone marrow appearances are those of megaloblastic anaemia. The nucleated red cells show an open nuclear chromatin pattern (most clearly seen on the high-power view of erythroblasts, **2d**). There are giant metamyelocytes in the white cell series (**2c, 2e**).

iii. The likeliest cause of megaloblastic anaemia in Crohn's disease is malabsorption of vitamin B_{12} due to disease of the terminal ileum.

A vitamin B_{12} absorption study gave the following results:

30 kBq of [^{58}Co]vitamin B_{12} and 18 kBq of [^{59}Co]vitamin B_{12} + Intrinsic Factor (IF) were given orally, together with 1 mg cyanocobalamin intramuscularly.
Her 24-hour urine volume was 1560 ml.
Dicopac Pt 1 – 3% of the dose was excreted in 24 hours (normal: 14–40%; in pernicious anaemia <10% ; in intestinal malabsorption <7%).
Dicopac Pt 2 – 3% of dose was excreted in 24 hours (normal: 14–40%; in pernicious anaemia >9%; in intestinal malabsorption <7%).
Excretion ratio – 1 (normal 0.7–1.2; in pernicious anaemia >1.3; in intestinal malabsorption 0.7–1.2).

This study demonstrates a failure of vitamin B_{12} absorption which is not corrected by administration of intrinsic factor. A radioactive carbon breath test would be a helpful further investigation, as it would exclude the presence of an intestinal stagnant loop with bacterial overgrowth.

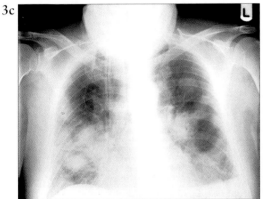

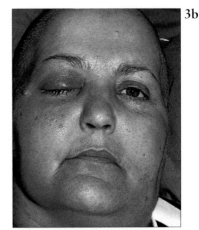

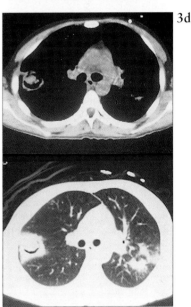

3 A 36-year-old female presented with a short history of increasing tiredness and bruising. Her blood count was as follows:

Hb	7.9 g/dl
WBC	34.8 x 10⁹/l
Platelets	21 x 10⁹/l

A bone marrow aspirate was taken (3a). Six weeks later, she developed a febrile illness with facial swelling and orbital oedema (3b). She also became short of breath and hypotensive, and had a single episode of haemoptysis. A chest X-ray (3c) and thoracic CT scan (3d) were performed.
i.   What is the presentation diagnosis?
ii. What is the likeliest cause of her febrile illness?
iii. How should she be treated?

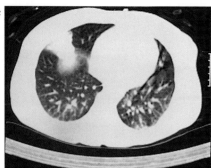

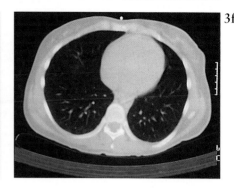

3 i. The bone marrow aspirate is infiltrated by primitive leukaemic cells which have Auer rods. The diagnosis is therefore acute myeloid leukaemia.

ii. Infection is clearly the likeliest cause in this setting. The marked facial cellulitis would be compatible with a Gram-positive skin infection but an X-ray of her sinuses should also be carried out. The chest X-ray shows widespread consolidation with ring shadows. Cavitation should be carefully looked for, and if present would support a diagnosis of staphylococcal pneumonia. The CT scan confirms cavitation, but the nature of these peripheral, triangular and enhancing lesions is highly suggestive of a fungal pneumonia.

iii. Every attempt must be made to make a microbiological diagnosis (blood cultures, culture of aspirate from skin, sputum culture, possibly bronchoalveolar lavage). She should receive broad-spectrum antibiotic and antifungal therapy, and this should include systemic amphotericin B.

The development of haemoptysis is disturbing, as there is a high risk of massive pulmonary haemorrhage in thrombocytopenic patients with invasive pulmonary fungal infections, and surgical resection should be considered for solitary lesions – this is probably inappropriate in this patient, who has multiple lesions.

Liposomal amphotericin is associated with a lower rate of renal toxicity, allowing higher doses (eg, 3 mg/kg/day) to be safely given. Figures **3e** and **3f** show thoracic CT scans in a leukaemic patient before and after therapy with liposomal amphotericin, demonstrating substantial resolution.

4 A 52-year-old woman with a previous history of carcinoma of the breast is admitted to hospital with a history of progressive bone pain.

i. Comment on the blood film appearances (**4a**).
ii. Comment on the bone marrow aspirate (**4b**).
iii. Comment on the bone marrow trephine (**4c**).
iv. What further tests are indicated?
v. What is the diagnosis?

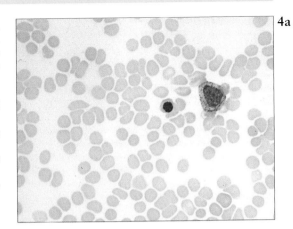

4a

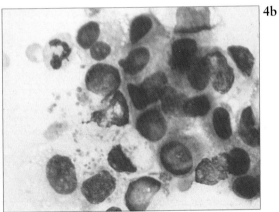

4b

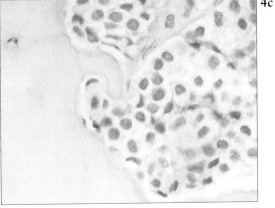

4c

4d

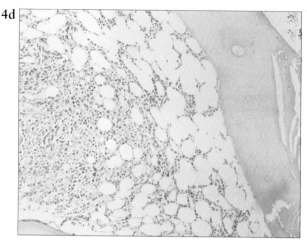

4e

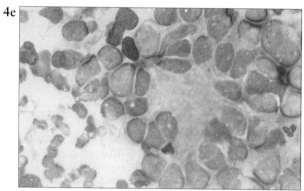

4 i. The blood film shows immature red and white blood cell forms, and is thus leukoerythroblastic. Possible causes are bone marrow infiltration, acute haemolysis, and overwhelming sepsis or bleeding – ie, situations in which the marrow is either replaced by abnormal cells (including fibrous tissue) or responding to an acute and overwhelming systemic illness.

ii. The marrow is infiltrated by abnormal, non-myeloid cells.

iii. Trephine biopsy confirms marrow infiltration.

iv. A bone scan will confirm secondary deposits. This patient may have hypercalcaemia (which can lead to renal failure) and the alkaline phosphatase (bone isoenzyme) may be raised. Immunocytochemistry may be used to confirm the origin of the infiltrating cells, eg, epithelial cells are usually positive for cytokeratin.

v. Carcinoma of the breast with bone marrow secondaries.

Other tumours that frequently affect the marrow include tumours of the bronchus (**4d**) prostate, renal and thyroid, and neuroblastoma in childhood (**4e**).

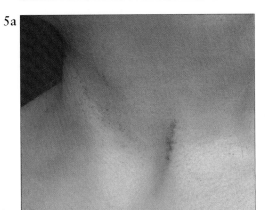

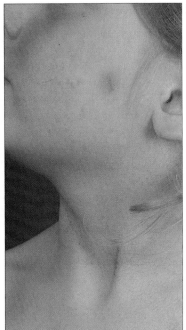

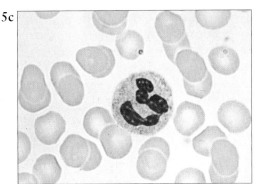

5 A 4-year-old child has a 3- to 4-day history of bruising over her face, neck and lower limbs. She has just recovered from a viral infection. Examination shows purpura over the legs and over her face (5a, 5b). The spleen is not palpable. Her blood count shows:

Hb	11.9 g/dl
WBC	9.3 x 10⁹/l (neutrophils 37%, lymphocytes 61%)
Platelets	9 x 10⁹/l
Prothrombin time	12 seconds (control 10–12 seconds)
APTT	35 seconds (control 30–40 seconds)
Fibrinogen	2.3 g/l (NR 2–4 g/l)
Creatinine	72 mmol/l

The blood film is shown (5c).

i. What is the likeliest diagnosis?
ii. What further tests are required?
iii. What treatment would you recommend?

5d

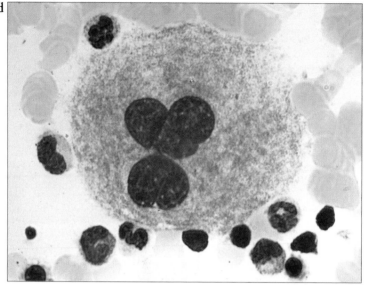

5 i. The blood film confirms thrombocytopenia, but there is no polychromasia, no red cell fragmentation and there is a normal neutrophil. The coagulation tests are normal, effectively excluding disseminated intravascular coagulation, and the creatinine is normal, excluding haemolytic uraemic syndrome. Immune thrombocytopenia (ITP) is the likeliest diagnosis.

ii. A bone marrow aspirate (5d) confirms the presence of megakaryocytes (large, multinuclear cells), thus suggesting platelet destruction. Platelet antibody testing is of much less value than the corresponding tests for red cells. An antinuclear factor assay should be performed. The preceding history of viral infection is consistent with ITP, though this is by no means universally seen.

iii. Avoidance of injury and antiplatelet drugs, eg, aspirin. The majority of children will recover spontaneously and need no therapy.

If the count does not recover spontaneously (eg, within 2 weeks) or if there is symptomatic bruising, particularly affecting mucous membranes such as the nose and mouth, then treatment is indicated. Prednisolone, starting at 0.5 mg/kg/day and reducing according to response, is the first-line therapy. Intravenous immunoglobulin (0.4 mg/kg/day) for 3–5 days is equally effective, but best reserved for non-responders. Splenectomy and other immunosuppressive drugs (eg, cyclophosphamide, azathioprine) are other possible approaches, but should be used cautiously in children.

Splenectomy is best avoided in children under five and should, in any event, be preceded by vaccination against pneumococcus and *Haemophilus influenzae* B, and followed by long-term oral penicillin V as prophylactic therapy against infection.

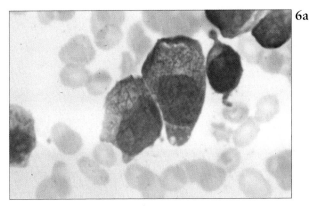

6a

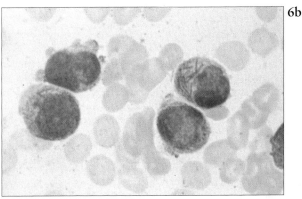

6b

6 A 36-year-old woman gives a 1-week history of tiredness. Her menstrual period has been going on for 10 days, and she has also noticed blood loss when brushing her teeth. Over the past day, she has developed a fever. Investigations show:

Hb	7.9 g/dl
WBC	3.2 x 10⁹/l
Platelets	11 x 10⁹/l
Prothrombin time	19 seconds (control 11–13 seconds)
APTT	64 seconds (control 30–40 seconds)
Thrombin time	28 seconds (control 18–20 seconds)
Fibrinogen	0.03 g/l (NR 2.0–4.0g/l)
Fibrin Degradation Product (FDP) titre	1:60 (NR <1:10)

i.   What abnormalities are seen on the blood film (6a) and bone marrow (6b)?
ii. What is the cause of the abnormal coagulation?
iii. What is the diagnosis?
iv. How is this condition managed?

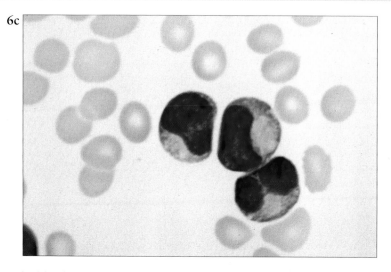

6 i. The blood and bone marrow film show leukaemic blast cells containing dense granules, many of which have condensed to form 'Auer' rods. Some cells have multiple Auer rods. This appearance is typical of acute promyelocytic leukaemia. This form of leukaemia is classified as M_3 and is usually associated with a translocation of material from chromosome 15 to chromosome 17 (t15–17). Figure 6c shows a variant form of M_3 (microgranular variant) where cytoplasmic granulation is less marked, but the 'dumb-bell' shaped nucleus is characteristic.

ii. The coagulation changes are consistent with disseminated intravascular coagulation.

iii. Acute promyelocytic leukaemia complicated by disseminated intravascular coagulation – a well-recognised association.

iv. The coagulopathy frequently gets worse when chemotherapy is commenced. There is great interest in the use of ATRA (*all-trans* retinoic acid), which can induce maturation of leukaemic cells, and its use is associated with a much lower incidence of disseminated intravascular coagulation. An intravenous infusion of heparin, with careful blood component therapy, will help to support the patient.

As with all forms of acute myeloid leukaemia, at least 3 courses of combination chemotherapy are required. Acute promyelocytic leukaemia has quite a good prognosis (approximately 40% cure rate with chemotherapy alone) but some haematologists would still recommend an allogeneic transplant if the patient has a histocompatible sibling.

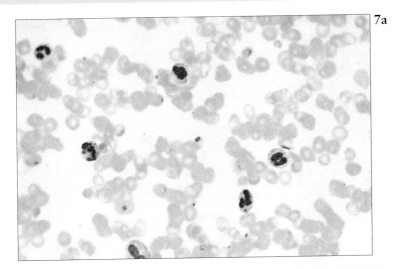

7a

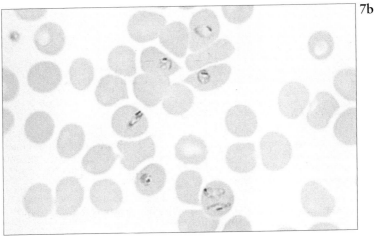

7b

7 i. What abnormality is seen on the blood film (7a, 7b)?
ii. What are the important haematological complications of this condition?
iii. What treatment should be offered?

7c 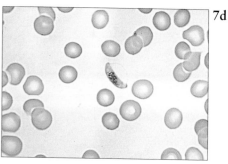 7d

7e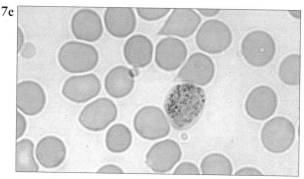

7 i. Malaria. The presence of more than one ring form per red cell strongly suggests *Plasmodium falciparum*.

ii. Anaemia, which is principally due to haemolysis of infected erythrocytes but is also due to immune haemolysis, splenomegaly, and impaired marrow production.

Thrombocytopenia is nearly always present, and is partly due to splenomegaly. Low-grade disseminated intravascular coagulation can also occur; this may be severe in overwhelming infection.

Leukopenia may arise from splenomegaly. Hypergammaglobulinaemia is frequent. Chronic malaria infection may lead to substantial splenomegaly ('tropical splenomegaly'), and the chronic immune stimulation may be a factor in the development of lymphoid malignancy (eg, lymphoma). Neutrophil leukocytosis and monocytosis may also occur.

iii. Falciparum malaria is commonly resistant to chloroquine, and is best treated with quinine (by intravenous infusion in severely ill patients). If quinine resistance is suspected, it should be followed by either fansidar or tetracycline. Mefloquine and halofantrine are also currently recommended for falciparum malaria.

Infections caused by *P. ovale*, *P. vivax* and *P. malariae* are usually less severe and chloroquine resistance is uncommon.

Figure 7c shows a mature schizont from a patient with *P. vivax* infection and 7d and 7e show gametes of *P. falciparum* and *P. vivax*, respectively.

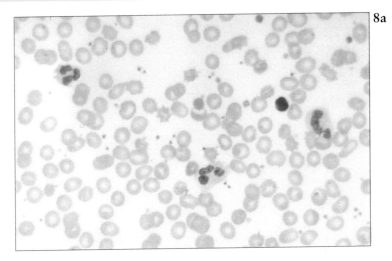

8a

8 A 34-year-old man has a history of chronic anaemia that was improved by an operation at the age of 11. He develops tiredness and shortness of breath after moderate exertion, but does not require blood transfusion and copes well with everyday activities. Drug therapy comprises folic acid 5 mg/day and penicillin V 250 mg twice daily. A full blood count shows:

Hb   8.5 g/dl
MCV   107 fl

i.   Comment on the blood film (8a).
ii. Comment on the following results of the autohaemolysis test. Haemolysis of red cells is assessed following incubation in isosmolar medium for 24 hours, with and without glucose.

	Without glucose	With glucose
Patient	7%	6.5%
Control	1.2%	0.2%
(NR)	0.1–3%	0.1–0.5%

iii. Suggest the likely diagnosis.

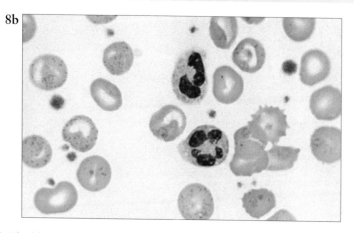

8b

8 i. The blood film shows irregularly contracted cells (pyknocytes) and target cells. A splenectomy is suggested, though the red cell abnormalities exceed those usually seen, simply as a result of splenectomy.

ii. The autohaemolysis test suggests an intrinsic red cell abnormality that leads to increased haemolysis. Glucose fails to correct the abnormality, suggesting that the defect involves the glycolytic pathway. An important differential diagnosis is hereditary spherocytosis, but the film does not show spherocytes and glucose usually partially corrects the membrane defect in haemoglobin.

iii. The commonest of the inherited glycolytic pathway enzymopathies, and the diagnosis in this case, is pyruvate kinase deficiency. Even so, this is a rare disease, with less than 300 cases reported world-wide.

The red cell lacks a nucleus and is unable to undertake protein synthesis to renew its supply of deficient enzymes; other tissues are able to compensate, though neurological and cardiac complications can occur with inherited red cell enzymopathies (eg, triose phosphate isomerase deficiency). The levels of 2,3 diphosphoglycerate (2,3 DGP) are usually elevated in patients with pyruvate kinase deficiency and this leads to improved oxygen delivery to tissues and better tolerance of anaemia.

Another cause of congenital haemolytic anaemia is the presence of an unstable haemoglobin variant (8b). These usually involve amino acid substitutions in the beta chain, though alpha and gamma chain variants are well described. Clinically, these disorders range from severe, with onset in early childhood, to mild, compensated haemolysis.

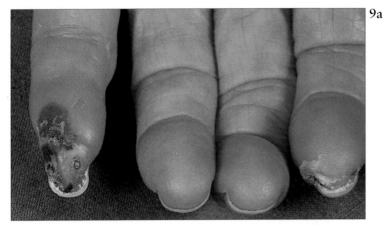

9a

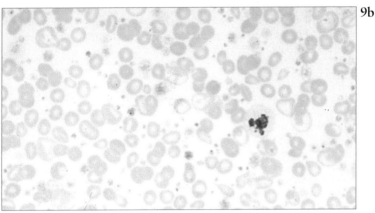

9b

9 A 76-year-old woman gives a 2–3 month history of progressively cold and numb fingertips. The symptoms are persistent but episodic. She is a non-smoker. Her feet are normal, and physical examination is otherwise unremarkable. All pulses are present. A blood count shows:

Hb	6 g/dl
WBC	14.6 x 10⁹/l (neutrophils 67%)
Platelets	1246 x 10⁹/l

Hb   6 g/dl
WBC   14.6 x 10^9/l (neutrophils 67%)
Platelets   1246 x 10^9/l

i. Comment on the patient's hands (9a).
ii. Comment on the blood film (9b).
iii. What are the causes of thrombocytosis?
iv. What further tests are warranted?
v. What treatment would you offer?

9c

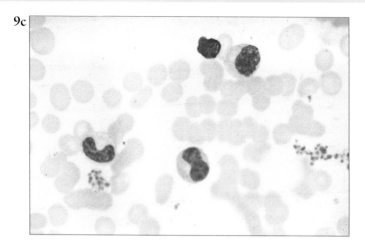

9 i. There are severe ischaemic changes affecting both hands.

ii. The blood film shows increased numbers of circulating platelets, with marked platelet anisocytosis and many giant platelets.

iii. Increased platelets may be primary or secondary. Primary thrombocythaemia turned out to be the diagnosis in this case, and this is a myeloproliferative disorder; a raised platelet count is also encountered as part of other myeloproliferative disorders, eg, chronic granulocytic leukaemia, polycythaemia vera. Secondary thrombocytosis occurs in response to infection, bleeding, iron deficiency and malignancy, and is seen after splenectomy.

iv. A full history and physical examination is needed to exclude causes of secondary thrombocytosis. A bone marrow aspirate and trephine biopsy may confirm primary thrombocythaemia. A serum ferritin is required to exclude iron deficiency, and abdominal ultrasound scan may detect splenomegaly. Platelet function tests are typically abnormal in primary thrombocythaemia and normal in secondary or reactive states.

v. Primary thrombocythaemia is treated with chemotherapy (eg, oral hydroxyurea) to lower the platelet count and maintain it below 400 x 10^9/l, and antiplatelet therapy (eg, aspirin 150 mg on alternate days) to inhibit platelet function.

Figure 9c shows increased platelet numbers in association with abnormal, hypogranular neutrophils. This patient had myelodysplasia; cytogenetic analysis showed the presence of 5q⁻, which is associated with a slowly progressive form of myelodysplasia with thrombocythaemia.

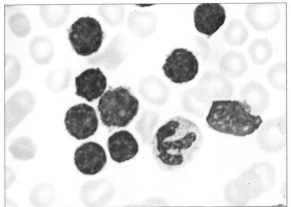

10a

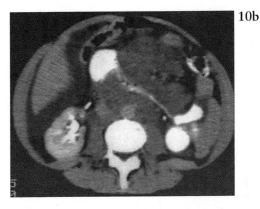

10b

10 A 76-year-old female was diagnosed 3 years ago as suffering from chronic lymphocytic leukaemia. She has not required any therapy, and was in good health until 4 weeks ago. She now complains of tiredness, polyuria and lethargy, and has also noticed increasing abdominal distension. On examination she is pale. She is not jaundiced, but she does have lymphadenopathy in both axillae. A marked swelling of the left elbow is noted. The spleen is easily palpable, and ascites is present. Neurological examination is normal.

i. Comment on the peripheral blood film findings (10a).
ii. Comment on the abdominal CT scan (10b).
iii. What is the likeliest diagnosis?

10c

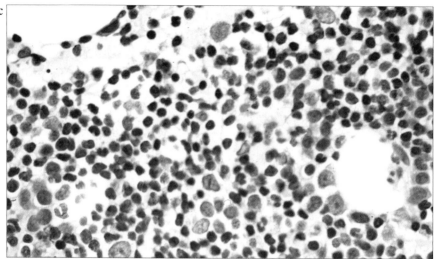

10d

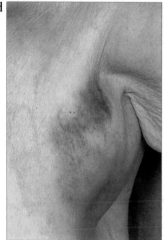

10 i. The film shows abnormal lymphoid cells which do not look like the mature B lymphocytes of chronic lymphocytic leukaemia. These are larger cells with nucleoli. These appearances are in keeping with an immunoblastic transformation of chronic lymphocytic leukaemia. The bone marrow trephine biopsy is shown in **10c**; it is hypercellular and heavily infiltrated by pleomorphic, large lymphocytes.

ii. The CT scan shows enlarged retroperitoneal lymph nodes. These are affecting the ureters, possibly causing ureteric obstruction, and they are perhaps also affecting the bowel. The history suggests she may be developing renal failure.

iii. Richter's syndrome denotes a transformation of chronic lymphocytic leukaemia into a more aggressive tumour, often with enlargement of lymph node tissue in unusual sites (eg, retroperitoneally). This patient also had massive axillary (**10d**) and epitrochlear nodes.

This condition responds poorly to therapy and is usually rapidly progressive.

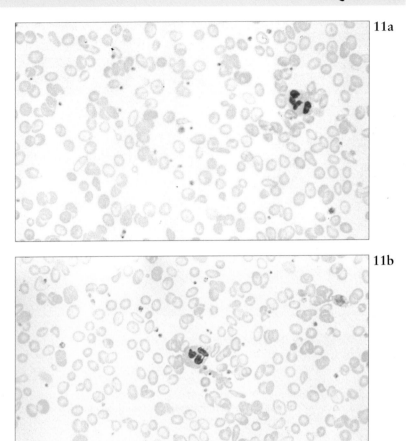

11a

11b

11 A 72-year-old woman presents with a 4–6 week history of gradually increasing tiredness and shortness of breath. A blood count shows:

Hb	8.6 g/dl
MCV	65 fl
MCH	26.4 pg
MCHC	29 g/dl
RBC	3.8 x 10¹²/l
WBC	6.7 x 10⁹/l (differential normal)
Platelets	456 x 10⁹/l

i.   What abnormalities are shown in the blood film (**11a, 11b**)?
ii. What is the diagnosis?
iii. What further investigations should be performed?

11c 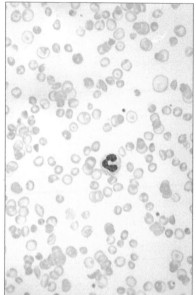 11d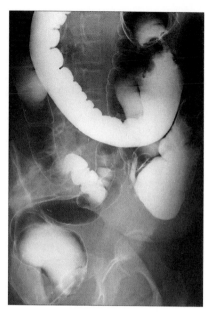

11 i. The blood count shows anaemia with microcytic, hypochromic red cell indices.
ii. The platelet count is raised, in keeping with iron deficiency anaemia. The blood film shows hypochromic, microcytic cells, with target cells, and increased and large platelet numbers.

The differential diagnosis of hypochromasia and microcytosis is thalassaemia. The carrier states for both alpha thalassaemia and beta thalassaemia are rarely associated with anaemia. Other causes of target cells include liver disease, post-splenectomy and other haemoglobinopathies, eg, haemoglobin C (**11c**).

iii. Investigations should aim at confirming iron deficiency and defining a cause. Serum iron is reduced, the iron-binding capacity is increased and the serum ferritin (which is an accurate measure of body iron stores) is reduced. The commonest cause of this picture is bleeding and, in a post-menopausal female or in a male, the cause of bleeding must be established.

In this patient, a barium enema (**11d**) was performed. This showed a carcinoma of the colon at the splenic flexure.

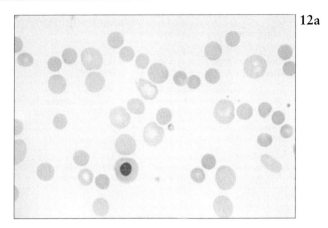

12a

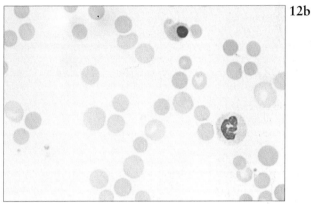

12b

12 A 6-year-old girl presents with a 4-week history of gradually increasing tiredness and lack of energy. She has also become jaundiced. There is no relevant past medical history. Examination reveals a pale, jaundiced child with no lymphadenopathy but with a spleen palpable 6 cm below the left costal margin. There are no signs of chronic liver disease. Cardiovascular examination reveals a soft apical systolic murmur. Investigations show:

Hb	6.1 g/dl
MCV	110 fl
Reticulocytes	22%
WBC	15.1 x 10⁹/l (neutrophils 12.3 x 10⁹/l)
Platelets	103 x 10⁹/l

i. What abnormalities are seen on the blood film (**12a, 12b**)?
ii. What is the likely diagnosis?
iii. What further investigations are indicated?
iv. How would you treat this patient?

12 i. The blood film shows polychromasia, anisocytosis, poikilocytosis and sphero-cytes, with circulating nucleated red blood cells.

ii. Auto-immune haemolytic anaemia.

iii. The direct antiglobulin test (DAT, Coomb's Test) is strongly positive, with complement and IgG detectable on the red cell surface.

Liver function tests show an elevated bilirubin (320 mmol/l) which is largely unconjugated. Her serum contains a pan-reacting red cell antibody that has no clear specificity and there is no evidence of an additional red cell alloantibody. The antibody reacts most strongly at 37°C.

Serum haptoglobin is often reduced and urine haemosiderin is present in the face of intravascular haemolysis.

An autoantibody screen reveals a positive antinuclear factor (ANF) at a titre of >1:100, suggesting underlying systemic lupus erythematosus (SLE).

An abdominal CT scan shows splenomegaly but no lymph node enlargement, and no evidence of an underlying lymphoma.

Red cell grouping and selection of blood for cross-matching should be done with care at an experienced laboratory.

iv. Prednisolone 1.0 mg/kg of body weight is first-line immunosuppression.

Splenectomy will reduce red cell destruction and also remove a site of autoantibody production. There is however an increased risk of infection postoperatively and the operation is best avoided in children under 5. Splenectomy must be preceded by pneumococcal and *H. influenzae* B vaccination and followed by long-term prophylactic penicillin. Second-line immunosuppressive therapy includes azathioprine, cyclophosphamide, cyclosporin and folic acid.

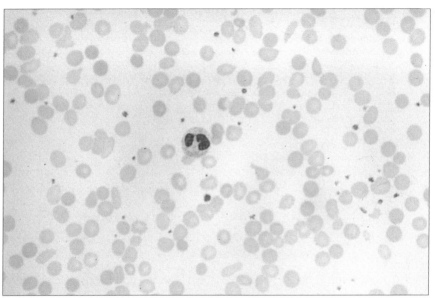

13a

13 The blood film (**13a**) is from a 35-year-old male who has the following blood count:

Hb   6.3 g/dl
MCV   81 fl
WBC   6.1 x 10⁹/l
Platelets   137 x 10⁹/l

i. What is the diagnosis?
ii. What is the pathogenesis of the anaemia?
iii. What other haematological complications may occur?

13b

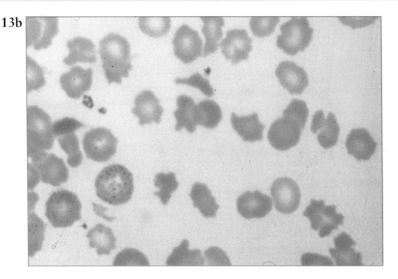

13 i. This patient is suffering from renal failure. The blood film shows characteristic echinocytes (Burr cells). The reticulocyte count is usually normal or slightly low, and bone marrow examination shows normoblastic erythropoiesis, often without the erythroid hyperplasia expected for the level of anaemia.

ii. The most important pathogenic mechanism is reduced production of erythropoietin by diseased kidneys. Treatment has been revolutionised by the availability of recombinant erythropoietin (EPO). Diminished red cell survival, iron deficiency through blood loss (eg, at haemodialysis) and secondary hyperparathyroidism are contributory factors.

iii. Other haematological complications of renal failure include:
- Polycythaemia, eg, following ectopic EPO production by renal tumours or cysts.
- Defects in platelet function, leading to a haemorrhagic diathesis partly correctable by DDAVP.
- Hypercoagulability, particularly in nephrotic syndrome, which is partly related to reduced fibrinolysis, reduced protein C, and reduced antithrombin III.
- Changes due to the underlying pathology causing renal failure (eg, auto-immune haemolytic anaemia and idiopathic thrombocytopenic purpura in systemic lupus erythematosus; low platelet count in disseminated intravascular coagulation).
- Treatment-induced changes (eg, immunosuppression).

Figure **13b** shows Burr cells and basophilic stippling in the blood film of another patient with renal failure.

14 A 22-year-old male complains of acute onset of generalised pains in the back, abdomen, and limbs. He has also had increased urinary frequency and pain in passing urine over the previous week. On examination he has a painful swelling of his right upper arm. His blood count shows:

Hb	8.4 g/dl
MCV	81 fl
WBC	33.4 x 10⁹/l
(neutrophils 86%)	
Platelets	390 x 10⁹/l

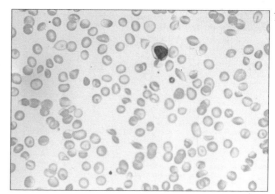

14a

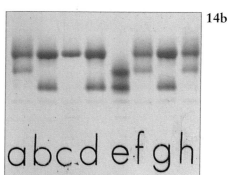

14b

i. What abnormalities are shown in the blood film (**14a**)?
ii. Haemoglobin electrophoresis was performed on the patient, his family, and controls (**14b**):

- Lane *a* is his mother.
- Lane *b* is his father.
- Lane *c* is his sister.
- Lane *d* is his brother.
- Lane *e* is the patient.
- Lane *f* is another brother.
- Lane *g* is a control sample of haemoglobin A/C blood.
- Lane *h* is a control of haemoglobin A/S blood.

What is the haematological diagnosis? Which of the siblings is likely to be symptomatic?
iii. What abnormality is on the X-ray (**14c**), and what complication has occurred?
iv. What other skeletal complications may occur?
v. What other renal complications may occur?

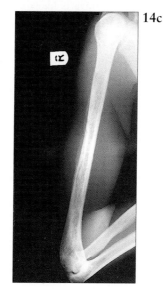

14c

14d

14e

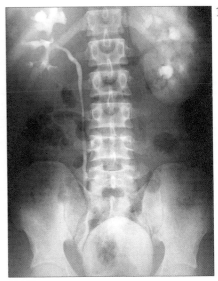

14 i. The blood film shows target cells and irregularly contracted red blood cells. Sickle cells are not prominent. Rectangular cells and cells in which the cytoplasm has shrunk away from the membrane are also seen.

ii. The findings in the blood film and the haemoglobin electrophoresis patterns suggest haemoglobin SC disease, the compound heterozygous state for the two important beta-chain mutants, haemoglobin S and C. None of the siblings has a significant haemoglobinopathy, and none of them is likely to be symptomatic. SC disease is a variant of homozygous sickle cell anaemia (SS disease) which is of almost equal severity and has a similar clinical presentation. This patient appears to have a sickle cell crisis which may have been preceded by a urinary tract infection.

iii. The X-ray (14c) shows sequestrum formation within the humerus. There is periosteal reaction. This suggests osteomyelitis. Blood culture revealed a bacteraemia with *Escherichia coli*, and the same organism was isolated from the right humerus. Patients with sickle cell anaemia have an increased risk of osteomyelitis, as organisms may enter the bloodstream from areas of mucosal damage (eg, in the urinary and gastrointestinal tracts) subjects are hyposplenic, and areas of infarcted marrow can be readily colonised by organisms. *Salmonella* osteomyelitis is particularly common, as hyposplenism predisposes to this organism, and bile from haemolysis within the marrow provides an enriched culture medium.

iv. The most important additional skeletal abnormality is avascular necrosis of the femoral head (14d) or the humeral head.

v. Renal papillary necrosis (14e) may occur in haemoglobin SC disease.

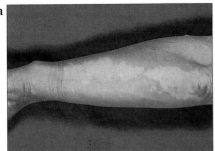

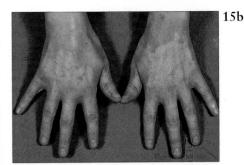

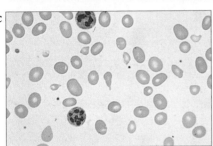

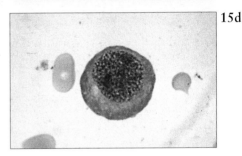

15 A 76-year-old woman presents with a 3–4 month history of gradually increasing tiredness and lethargy. She has also noticed numbness and tingling of the hands. On examination she is pale and slightly icteric. A skin rash is noted (15a). Sensory testing of the legs shows diminished sensation affecting both feet symmetrically. Both ankle jerks are absent and the knee jerks are brisk. A blood count shows:

Hb	6.5 g/dl
MCV	110 fl
WBC	2.5 x 10⁹/l
Platelets	103 x 10⁹/l

i. What is the dermatological diagnosis (15a, 15b)?
ii. What is the haematological diagnosis (15c, 15d)? What abnormalities are shown on the blood film?
iii. What is the neurological diagnosis?
iv. What further investigations are warranted?
v. How should the patient be treated?

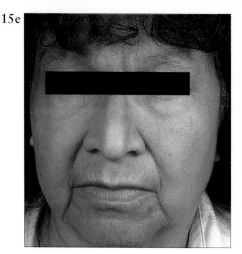

15e

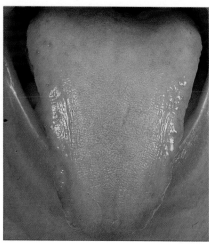

15f

15 **i.** Vitiligo. This is associated with organ-specific auto-immune diseases, eg,
• Pernicious anaemia.
• Thyroid disease.
• Addison's disease.
• Hypoparathyroidism.
ii. Pernicious anaemia. The blood film shows macrocytosis, anisocytosis and hyper-segmented polymorphonuclear leukocytes. There is also a circulating megaloblast. Deficiency of vitamin B_{12} is caused by failure of absorption of the vitamin. Antibodies to gastric parietal cells are present in 95% of patients with pernicious anaemia, but only 10% of normal individuals. Antibodies to intrinsic factor are found in 60% of people with pernicious anaemia.
iii. Subacute combined degeneration of the spinal cord, with a characteristic combination of upper and lower motor neuron signs in the legs.
iv. The following investigations should be carried out:
• Serum $B_{12.}$
• Serum folate and ferritin, and red cell folate (a reduced red cell folate with raised serum folate is characteristically seen in B_{12} deficiency).
• TSH level.
• A study of B_{12} absorption (eg, Schilling test).
An upper gastrointestinal endoscopy is advised.
v. Administration of folic acid without B_{12} therapy can lead to worsening of the neurological changes.
   Parenteral B_{12} – hydroxycobalamin 1000 mg intramuscularly weekly for 4 weeks followed by long-term injections every 3 months – is appropriate. Iron and folate supplements should be given orally for the first 2 months of treatment.
   Figure **15e** shows facial pallor with mild jaundice ('lemon-yellow tinge') in a woman with PA who has dyed her hair (premature greying is characteristic). Figure **15f** shows her fleshy tongue. These patients have an increased incidence of gastric carcinoma.

16a 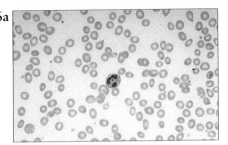 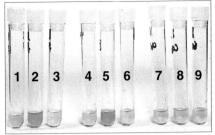 16b

16 A 56-year-old woman has noticed increasing tiredness and malaise. She was intensively investigated for iron deficiency 1 year ago and no cause was found. She has subsequently noticed episodes of pain associated with passage of dark urine. Investigations show:

Hb	9.5 g/dl
MCV	72 fl
WBC	41.7 x 10⁹/l
Platelets	113 x 10⁹/l

i. Comment on the blood film (16a) and blood count.
ii. A specialised test (16b) is performed on her serum and cells. There are 9 tubes, as follows :
1. Patient cells with patient serum (unacidified).
2. Patient cells with patient serum (acidified).
3. Patient cells with patient serum (acidified and heated).
4. Patient cells with donor serum (unacidified).
5. Patient cells with donor serum (acidified).
6. Patient cells with donor serum (acidified and heated).
7. Donor cells with donor serum (unacidified).
8. Donor cells with donor serum (acidified).
9. Donor cells with donor serum (acidified and heated).
iii. What is the diagnosis?
iv. What is the pathogenesis and natural history of this disease?

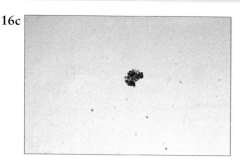 16c

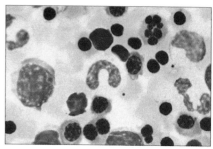 16d

16 i. The blood film shows hypochromic microcytic red cells which are consistent with iron deficiency. There is a disproportionate degree of anisocytosis and polychromasia.

ii. This is an illustration of Ham's test, and demonstrates that her red cells have increased sensitivity to lysis by complement present in her own serum.

Heat inactivates complement, whereas low pH activates complement. Thus, lysis of her cells occurs to a small extent in the presence of her own serum and donor serum, is exaggerated by the presence of acidified serum, and does not occur when complement is inactivated. Donor cells do not undergo lysis, and would not do so even in the presence of the patient's serum. The intravascular haemolysis leads to the presence of haemosiderin, which can be stained by Perl's reaction (**16c**) on the urine deposit. The only other disorder that may give a positive Ham's test is a rare congenital dyserythropoietic anaemia (CDA type II, HEMPAS – hereditary erythrocyte multinuclearity with positive acidified serum test, **16d**).

HEMPAS cells carry an unusual antigen that reacts with a lytic antibody present in about 30% of normal sera; lysis would not occur in tube 2, but may occur in tubes 4 and 5.

iii. Paroxysmal nocturnal haemoglobinuria (PNH).

iv. This is an acquired clonal disorder of the haemopoietic stem cell characterised by defects in the cell membrane which lead to impaired inactivation of complement, and thus to increased complement-mediated lysis. Many patients have defective platelet function and a thrombotic tendency, and presentation with hepatic vein thrombosis (Budd–Chiari syndrome) is well recognised.

Patients with PNH may develop pancytopenia with aplastic anaemia, and a proportion go on to develop acute myeloid leukaemia. Supportive therapy with blood transfusion is frequently required. The transfused cells should be filtered to remove contaminating leukocytes, as the transfusion of such leukocytes may lead to sensitization to HLA antigens, which can lead to complement activation and further haemolysis.

The basic defect in PNH probably involves a mutation in a gene encoding an anchor protein on the cell surface; this protein probably has a role in complement activation and signal transduction across the cell surface.

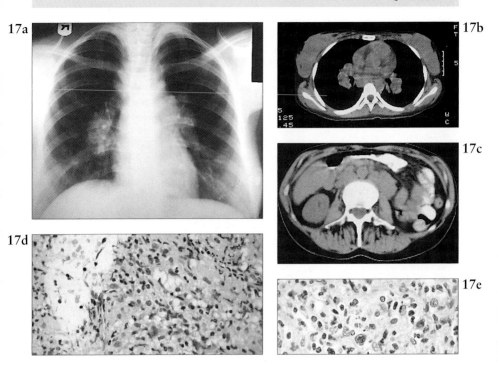

17 A 41-year-old male has a 6-week history of fever and night sweats. He has lost 2 kg in weight. He has had a recent cough with productive sputum, but his fever has failed to subside after a course of antibiotics. He smokes 10 cigarettes a day and drinks 16 units of alcohol a week. On examination he is pale and looks unwell. There is no palpable lymphadenopathy or splenomegaly. Investigation show:

Hb	8.7 g/dl	MCV	81 fl
Platelets	310 x 10⁹/l	ESR	91 mm/hour
Urea and electrolytes	normal	Immunoglobulins	normal
WBC	9.1 x 10⁹/l (differential normal)		
Bilirubin	61 mmol/l (NR 5–17 mmol/l)		
AST	137 U/l (NR 5–40 U/l)		
Alkaline phosphatase	250 U/l (NR 35–130 U/l)		
GGT	215 U/l (NR 10–48 U/l)		
Albumin	34 g/l (NR 35–50 g/l)		

i.   Comment on the chest X-ray (**17a**) and the thoracic CT scan (**17b**).
ii. Comment on the abdominal CT scan (**17c**).
iii. A laparotomy with splenectomy, liver biopsy (**17d**), and lymph node biopsy is performed. A bone marrow aspirate and trephine (**17e**) are also performed. Comment on the liver biopsy (**17d**). Comment on the bone marrow biopsy (**17e**).
iv. What is the diagnosis?
v.   How should he be treated?

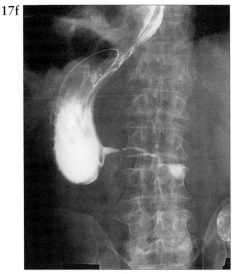 17f

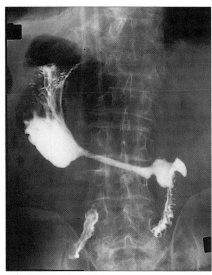 17g

17 i. The chest X-ray shows a large mediastinal mass, compatible with lymph node enlargement.

ii. Abdominal CT scan shows enlargement of the retroperitoneal lymph nodes between the junction of the renal vessels and the bifurcation of the aorta.

iii. The liver biopsy shows infiltration of the liver by large multinucleated cells which have the appearance of Reed–Sternberg cells. Bone marrow trephine shows an abnormal area at one end of the core which, at high power, also reveals involvement by Hodgkin's disease.

iv. Stage IVB mixed cellularity Hodgkin's disease.

v. Localised Hodgkin's disease (eg, stages I and IA) responds well to radiotherapy.

However, systemic symptoms, involvement of tissues both above and below the diaphragm (Stage III) and involvement extending outside the lymphoreticular system (eg, into the liver, marrow, lung, central nervous system, skin – Stage IV) should be treated with combination chemotherapy. Suitable regimes are MOPP (mustine, vincristine [Oncovin] procarbazine, prednisolone), ChlVPP (chlorambucil, vinblastine, procarbazine, prednisolone) and ABVD (adriamycin, BCNU, vinblastine, dacarbazine).

Side effects of combination chemotherapy include bone marrow suppression, hair loss, susceptibility to infection, and infertility. There is an increased risk of acute myeloid leukaemia in lymphoma patients who have received combination chemotherapy, particularly if they have also received radiotherapy.

Figure **17f** shows gastric involvement and pyloric obstruction by high grade non Hodgkin's lymphoma; barium flow and symptoms were both improved by radiotherapy (**17g**).

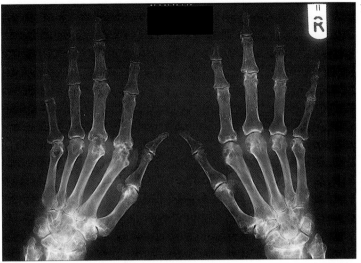

18a

18 A 56-year-old woman, with a long history of arthritis, has an abnormal blood count:

Hb	9.1 g/dl
MCV	79 fl
MCHC	32.1
WBC	7.2 x 10⁹/l
Platelets	195 x 10⁹/l

i. What diagnosis is suggested by the X-ray of her hands (18a)?
ii. What is the likeliest cause of her anaemia?
iii. What investigations would you perform on this patient?
iv. What other haematological complications may occur in this condition?

18b

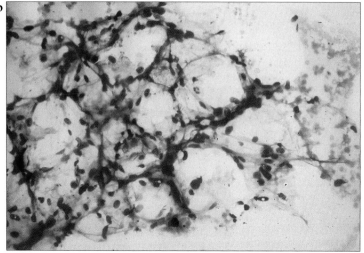

18 i. The X-ray confirms the diagnosis of rheumatoid arthritis – it shows an erosive arthritis affecting her hands.

ii. The anaemia of chronic disease (ACD). This normochromic normocytic (occasionally slightly microcytic) anaemia commonly complicates chronic inflammatory and infective conditions and neoplasia. The mechanism is poorly understood but it probably involves a suppressive effect that increased cytokine levels (eg, tumour necrosis factor, interleukin 6) have on erythropoiesis, the release of iron from the reticuloendothelial system, and iron utilisation.

iii. The serum iron and the total iron-binding capacity are typically lowered in ACD.
  The serum ferritin is usually normal, though it may be raised in the face of active inflammation. A lowered serum ferritin would suggest iron deficiency, which frequently complicates rheumatoid arthritis (eg, due to gastric bleeding induced by ingestion of non-steroidal anti-inflammatory drugs). Vitamin B_{12} and folic acid levels, thyroid function, renal function, liver function and ESR would be worth assessing.

iv. Other haematological complications of rheumatoid arthritis include:
• Immunological disorders – auto-immune haemolytic anaemia, idiopathic thrombocytopenic purpura, leukopenia, Felty's syndrome (leukopenia and splenomegaly).
• Therapy-induced complications – gastrointestinal bleeding, cytopenias, aplastic anaemia (caused, for example, by phenylbutazone); **18b** shows a fragment of a bone marrow aspirate taken from a patient with phenylbutazone-induced aplastic anaemia.
• An increased incidence of lymphoma.
• Amyloidosis.

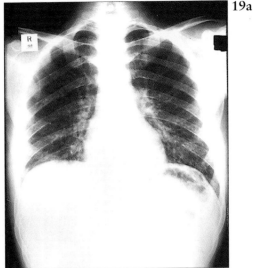

19a

19 A 34-year-old patient, with a past history of intravenous drug abuse, presents with a 7-day history of progressive shortness of breath. On examination he is pyrexial and has clear dyspnoea and tachycardia. His blood pressure is reduced at 90/60. Oxygen saturation when breathing 40% oxygen is reduced at 86%, and he is sweating. His full blood count shows:

Hb	8.5 g/dl
WBC	17.5 x 10⁹/l (neutrophils 79%)
Platelets	105 x 10⁹/l

i. What is the likeliest diagnosis from the history and chest X-ray (19a)?
ii. What further tests should be performed?
iii. How should he be treated?
iv. What other haematological complications may occur in this condition?

19b

19c

19d

19e

19 i. He probably has infection with *Pneumocystis carinii*.

ii. HIV antibody. A bronchoalveolar lavage or bronchial secretions should be obtained so that a firm microbiological diagnosis can be made; this should done after consultation with an anaesthetist. He needs to be assessed for admission to an intensive therapy unit. A full biochemical screen should be performed, and blood, urine and a throat swab should be sent for bacterial, viral, fungal and protozoan culture.

iii. He should be treated with high-dose intravenous co-trimoxazole for presumed *Pneumocystis* infection, but broad-spectrum antibiotics should be given until a bacteriological diagnosis is proven and in case of mixed infections. High-dose co-trimoxazole may cause myelosuppression, partly reversible with folinic acid.

iv. Immune thrombocytopenia, lymphopenia and anaemia of chronic disease are relatively common. Monocytosis, a haemophagocytic syndrome, immune haemolytic anaemia, and aplastic anaemia are also reported.

The blood film (**19b**) is from an HIV-positive patient who is on zidovudine; it shows macrocytosis and thrombocytopenia. There is an increased incidence of lymphoma, especially high-grade B cell lymphoma (as illustrated in the bone marrow aspirate, **19c**).

Myelodysplasia and acute leukaemia are reported. A Ziehl–Nielson stain on a bone marrow trephine biopsy in an HIV-positive patient (**19d**) shows multiple organisms, which on culture were confirmed to be *Mycobacterium avium intracellulare*. Bone marrow trephine biopsy in an HIV positive patient (**19e**) shows infection with *Cryptococcus neoformans*.

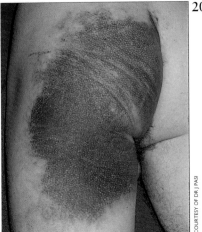

20a

COURTESY OF DR. J. PASI

20 A male child (20a) presents with excessive bleeding following a fall while riding his bicycle. He has not had surgery previously, but his mother reveals that he does bleed easily and that he bleeds excessively following cuts and abrasions. There is no relevant family history. Physical examination is normal. Tests show:

Hb	9.7 g/dl
WBC	12.9 x 10⁹/l (neutrophils 67%)
Platelets	310 x 10⁹/l
PT	11 seconds (control 11–13 seconds)
APTT	>120 seconds (control 30–40 seconds)
Thrombin time	18 seconds (control 18–20 seconds)
APTT with 50:50 mix with normal plasma	55 seconds (control 30–40 seconds)

i. What is the likely diagnosis?
ii. What further investigations are required?
iii. How should this condition be treated?

20 i. The history and finding of a prolonged APTT which shows partial correction by addition of normal plasma suggests an inherited bleeding tendency within the intrinsic pathway of the coagulation cascade. These findings would be compatible with:

• Haemophilia A (factor VIII deficiency).
• Haemophilia B (Christmas disease, factor IX deficiency).
• Von Willebrand's disease (factor VIII-related antigen, VIII RAG, von Willebrand factor deficiency).

Factor XI deficiency could also cause these changes: this is commonest in Jewish populations and is often asymptomatic. The history (but not the APTT results) would be consistent with a defect of platelet function.
ii. Factor VIII level was 1.5% (NR 50–150%), and factor VIII RAG was 78% (NR 50–150%), confirming that this patient has factor VIII deficiency of moderate severity. Approximately one-third of patients have a new mutation and no family history. Both haemophilia A and B are X-linked (ie, the genes for factors VIII and IX are encoded on the X chromosome) and family members should be screened, because the mother and sisters may be carriers and male siblings may have the disease. Plasma should be routinely screened for the presence of a factor VIII inhibitor, though such inhibitors are usually present only after treatment with clotting factor concentrates.
iii. Treatment is best conducted at a haemophilia centre with full laboratory, clinical and community services. Current guidelines favour the use of high-purity, heat-treated factor VIII concentrate for treatment of bleeding episodes and prophylaxis at times of surgery. Recombinant factor VIII is now available. An important complication of earlier therapy with concentrates that had not been heat-treated was transmission of viral infections such as HIV and hepatitis C.

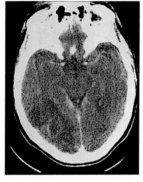

21a

21b

21 A 68-year-old man presents with a 12-hour history of headache, confusion and declining consciousness. His wife says he has recently completed oral chemotherapy for an 'indolent form of leukaemia'. Examination reveals him to be responding to painful stimuli but not to verbal commands. He has bilateral axillary and inguinal lymphadenopathy. He is clinically jaundiced and anaemic. His spleen is palpably enlarged. He has neck stiffness, generalised hyper-reflexia and bilateral upgoing plantar reflexes. Fundal examination is normal, and there are no focal neurological signs. Full blood count shows:

Hb	7.5 g/dl
WBC	37 x 10⁹/l (lymphocytes 86%)
Platelets	26 x 10⁹/l

i. What abnormalities are seen on this patient's blood film (**21a**)?
ii. Suggest a possible haematological diagnosis.
iii. What abnormalities are seen on the enhanced CT scan (**21b**)?
iv. How should this patient be managed ?

21 i. The film shows spherocytosis, polychromasia, thrombocytopenia, and lymphocytosis.
ii. The 'indolent form of leukaemia' in this case was chronic lymphocytic leukaemia (CLL), which became complicated by auto-immune haemolytic anaemia. (This is a recognised association.) Direct antiglobulin test, reticulocyte count, lymphoid cell immunephenotype analysis and bone marrow examination are required to confirm this. Immune phenotype analysis will show these cells to be positive for B cell markers [CD 19, 20, 21 and 23] and to have low density of surface membrane immunoglobulin [SmIg] with predominance of one light chain, either kappa or lambda. B-CLL cells also characteristically and aberrantly express the T cell marker, CD5.
iii. The scan shows a low attenuation area in the right parieto-occipital area. There is no evidence of midline shift. This is not consistent with acute bleeding, but suggests infection–inflammation or infarction.
iv. He requires urgent lumbar puncture. In this case, it showed intracellular Gram-positive rods, consistent with *Listeria* meningitis. The low platelet count suggests possible disseminated intravascular coagulation (DIC), which frequently complicates meningitis.

He was treated with intravenous ampicillin, chloramphenicol and metronidazole. His auto-immune haemolytic anaemia responded to high-dose intravenous steroids (dexamethasone was chosen to reduce cerebral oedema) and blood transfusion.

22 i. Comment on the abnormalities in the blood film (**22a, 22b**). The patient's blood count shows:

Hb	9.1 g/dl
MCV	62 fl
WBC and platelets	normal

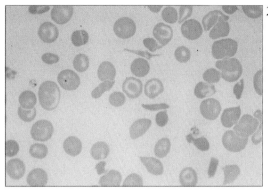

22a

ii. Haemoglobin electrophoresis (**22c**) has been performed on:
• The patient (lane *f*).
• His mother (lane *e*).
• His father (lane *d*).

Appropriate controls as follows:
• Lane *a*: beta thalassaemia trait.
• Lane *b*: sickle cell trait.
• Lane *c*: normal.

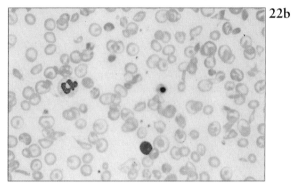

22b

Quantification of separated haemoglobin bands in the patient shows:
• Hb F   9%
• Hb S   86%
• Hb A$_2$ 5%

Quantification of separated haemoglobin bands in his mother shows:
• Hb F   3% (NR <1%)
• Hb A   92%
• Hb A$_2$ 5% (NR 1.5–3.5%)

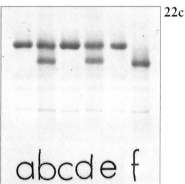

22c

Quantification of separated haemoglobin bands in his father shows:
• Hb A   47%
• Hb S   49%
• Hb A$_2$ 3%

What is the diagnosis in the patient? What is the diagnosis in his mother and his father?

iii. The patient has decided to marry someone who is a sickle cell trait carrier. What advice would you give?

22d

Disease	Origin →	A₂	C	S	F	A
Normal	|	|			|	■
Sickle cell trait	|	|		■	|	■
Sickle cell disease	|	|		■	|	
Sickle-C	|	|	■	■	|	
C-trait	|	|	■		|	■
Thalassemia major	|				■	|
Thalassemia minor	|	■			|	■
Sickle-thalassemia	|	■		■	|	|

22 i. The blood film shows hypochromic, microcytic cells with target cells and occasional sickle cells. These appearances are consistent with sickle beta thalassaemia.

ii. The patient has sickle beta thalassaemia. The patient's mother has beta thalassaemia trait. His father has sickle cell trait. By cellulose acetate (alkaline pH) electrophoresis (22c), Hb C migrates to the same position as Hb A_2. Agar gel electrophoresis allows separation of Hb C and Hb A_2. Figure 22d illustrates the expected pattern of migration of normal and abnormal haemoglobins by cellulose acetate (alkaline pH) electrophoresis in a diagrammatic form. Hb A is composed of 2 alpha chains and 2 beta chains ($\alpha_2\beta_2$); Hb A_2 is composed of 2 alpha chains and 2 delta chains ($\alpha_2\delta_2$); Hb F is 2 alpha chains and 2 gamma chains ($\alpha_2\gamma_2$). Patients with beta thalassaemia have impaired production of beta chains and compensate by increasing their production of Hb A_2 and Hb F.

iii. The patient has S/β thal and the partner is denoted A/S. The possible combinations for their offspring are therefore:

• S/A.
• S/S.
• A/β thal.
• beta thal/S.

There is thus a 50% chance of a significant haemoglobinopathy (S/S or S/beta thal). These two conditions have a similar clinical presentation and course. Non-directional, informed counselling should be offered to the couple. Antenatal diagnosis may be offered, with the prospect of genetic diagnosis by DNA analysis of placental tissue at 8–12 weeks of pregnancy.

23 i. This blood film (**23a**, **23b**) is from a 34-year-old woman who has a WBC of 63 x 10⁹/l. She is treated with four courses of intensive chemotherapy and enters complete remission. She then receives an allogeneic bone marrow transplant from a fully HLA compatible sibling. She recovers from the procedure but 9 weeks later she develops increasing shortness of breath. Her chest X-ray is shown in **23c**.

ii. What is the differential diagnosis and how would you manage her?

iii. What is the pathogenesis of this condition?

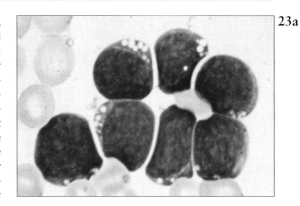

23a

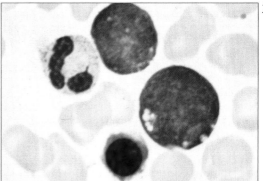

23b

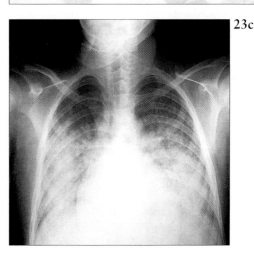

23c

23 i. The blood film shows large numbers of blast cells with intensely basophilic cytoplasm and vacuoles. These features suggest B cell acute lymphoblastic leukaemia, but an identical appearance is seen in Burkitt's lymphoma. The cells are positive for the presence of monoclonal surface-membrane immunoglobulin.

ii. Nearly all patients have a chromosomal translocation involving the c-*myc* onco-gene (chromosome 8) and one of the loci for immunoglobulin genes (typically the heavy chain locus on chromosome 14). It seems likely that this event is involved in the abnormal and uncontrolled proliferation of primitive B lymphocytes seen in this condition.

Burkitt's lymphoma typically occurs in African children, who have chronic B cell stimulation as a result of malaria endemicity. Most of these children also have evidence of recent infection by the B lymphotropic virus, Epstein–Barr virus. Although t(8;14) is the commonest translocation, variant forms include t(2;8) and t(8;22).

iii. She has developed bilateral diffuse pulmonary infiltrates in association with dysp-noea. Non-infectious causes, eg, pulmonary oedema, chemotherapy toxicity and pulmonary haemorrhage, are commoner in the first post-transplant month. However at 9 weeks an infectious cause is more likely (eg, viral – CMV, herpes simplex, varicella zoster, respiratory syncytial virus), *Pneumocystis carinii* (though the use of routine co-trimoxazole or pentamadine prophylaxis has made this less common) and fungal or bacterial infection. CMV seronegative bone marrow transplant recipients should receive CMV negative blood components.

Blood gas/oxygen saturation analysis and clinical review by an ITU physician are mandatory. An accurate microbiological diagnosis should be sought, eg, by bron-choalveolar lavage with possible transbronchial biopsy, sputum culture and cytology, blood, tissue and urine cultures particularly for CMV (eg, by DEAFF test – detection of early antigen fluorescent foci or polymerase chain reaction), and CT scan for evidence of fungal or pneumocystis infection.

Empirical broad-spectrum antibiotic and anti-viral therapy (eg, IV ganciclovir plus CMV hyper-immune globulin) are required and specific anti-pneumocystis (with high dose co-trimoxazole) and anti-fungal therapy (with IV amphotericin) should be considered.

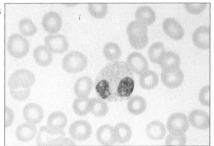

24a

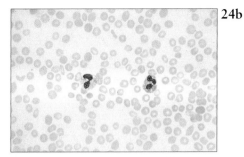

24b

24 A 37-year-old woman of African origin is diagnosed as suffering from tuberculosis. Treatment is commenced with isoniazid (in combination with pyridoxine), rifampicin and ethambutol. After 2 weeks on this regime, she develops bruising over her legs. A full blood count shows

Hb	11.1 g/dl
WBC	11.7 x 10⁹/l
(neutrophils 9.0 x 10⁹/l, lymphocytes 1.8 x 10⁹/l, eosinophils 0.9 x 10⁹/l)	
Platelets	6 x 10⁹/l

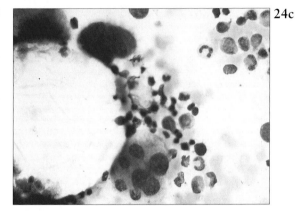

24c

A bone marrow aspirate is performed.

i. Comment on the appearance of the blood film (**24a, 24b**) and the bone marrow aspirate (**24c, 24d**).

ii. Why does she have bruising?

iii. Why is she on pyridoxine?

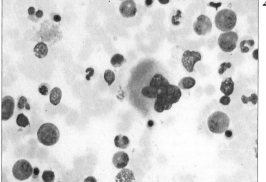

24d

24e

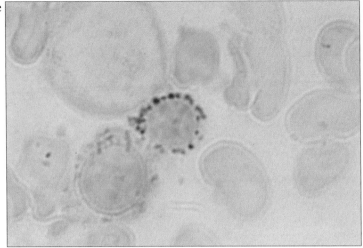

24 i. The blood film shows eosinophils, which may indicate drug allergy. The bone marrow aspirate shows megakaryocytes, and eosinophil precursors are also evident.
ii. She has thrombocytopenia. The presence of megakaryocytes in the marrow suggests that platelet production is adequate and destruction must be increased. Immune destruction of platelets is well recognised as a complication of rifampicin. Other drugs that can have this effect include heparin, sulphonamides, and thiazide diuretics. Thrombocytopenia can also occur because of a drug-induced decreased platelet production (eg, chemotherapeutic and immunosuppressive drugs).
iii. Isoniazid therapy can cause sideroblastic anaemia by antagonising the action of pyridoxine (vitamin B_6), thus disturbing haem synthesis. **24e** is an iron stain of bone marrow and shows abnormal iron granules in a perinuclear location (ringed sideroblasts). Hence it is important to give pyridoxine supplements with isoniazid.

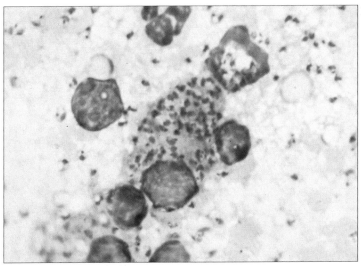
25a

25 A 31-year-old woman returned 3 months ago from a long holiday in the Middle East and North Africa, where she travelled widely and slept in a tent or in cheap hotels. She gives a 2-week history of fever, anorexia and abdominal discomfort. She has taken malaria prophylaxis. There is no history of diarrhoea or constipation. On examination she is pale but not jaundiced. There is no lymphadenopathy, but the spleen is palpable 8 cm below the left costal margin, and the liver is also clinically enlarged. Investigations show:

Hb	9.3 g/dl
WBC	3.4 x 10⁹/l (lymphocytes 40%, neutrophils 55%)
Platelets	74 x 10⁹/l
Urea and electrolytes	normal
Liver function tests	normal
Stool, blood, urine, throat saliva culture	negative

A liver biopsy (**25a**) was performed.
i. What is the diagnosis?
ii. What other features may occur in this condition?
iii. What is the recommended therapy?

25b

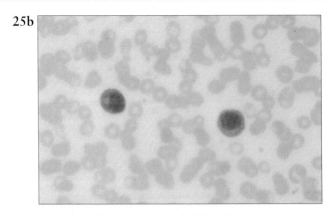

25c

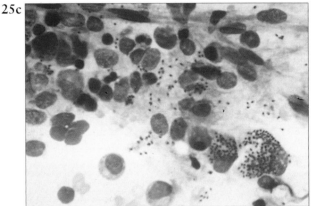

25 i. The liver biopsy (**25a**) shows Leishman–Donovan bodies within a macrophage, and the diagnosis is visceral Leishmaniasis (kala-azar). Her mild pancytopenia is due to splenic enlargement, though a mild leukopenia can also occur as part of the disease.

ii. Infection with *Leishmania donovani*, which is a protozoan, is transmitted by the bite of sandflies, typically from an animal (eg, dog) reservoir. The reservoir is humans in the Indian form of the disease. Hepatosplenomegaly, sometimes with lymphopenia, is typically seen. Hypergammaglobulinaemia, notably a polyclonal increase in IgM, and a correspondingly raised ESR are other noteworthy features. The peripheral blood film (**25b**) showed circulating, reactive plasma cells and rouleaux. Leishman-Donovan bodies are also seen in the bone marrow aspirate (**25c**).

iii. Pentavalent antimonials, eg, sodium stibogluconate, are the drugs of choice.

26 A 75-year-old woman presented with a 3-month history of gradually increasing tiredness. She had generalised lymphadenopathy. Abdominal examination revealed a palpable spleen 8 cm below the left costal margin. A blood count showed:

Hb	8.9 g/dl
WBC	23.7 x 10⁹/l
(lymphocytes 81%,	
neutrophils 18%)	
Platelets	109 x 10⁹/l

Hb 8.9 g/dl
WBC 23.7 x 10^9/l
(lymphocytes 81%, neutrophils 18%)
Platelets 109 x 10^9/l

i. Comment on the blood film (**26a**).
ii. Comment on the bone marrow trephine biopsy (**26b**).
iii. What is the differential diagnosis?
iv. The patient developed profound hypothermia and sleepiness 2 years later. There were no focal neurological signs. A CT scan of the brain was performed (**26c**). What complication has occurred?

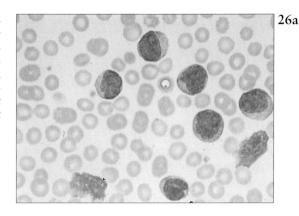

26a

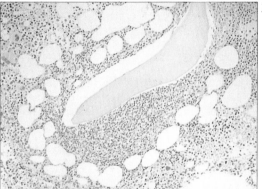

26b

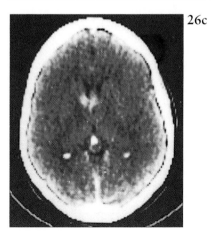

26c

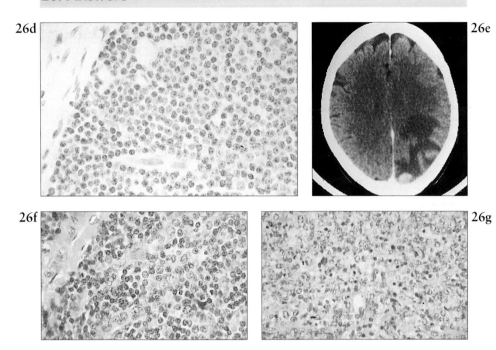

26d

26e

26f

26g

26 i. The film shows circulating atypical lymphoid cells with cleaved nuclei. The mild thrombocytopenia is due to splenomegaly. The count also shows a lymphocytosis.

ii. The biopsy shows abnormal deposits of mature lymphoid cells along the bony trabeculae – so-called paratrabecular deposits.

iii. This patient has a chronic lymphoproliferative disorder. The likeliest diagnosis is low-grade follicular lymphoma, confirmed by lymph node biopsy (**26d**). Other possibilities would include chronic lymphocytic leukaemia and its variants (hairy cell leukaemia, splenic lymphoma with villous lymphocytes, prolymphocytic leukaemia).Cytogenetic analysis showed translocation t(14;18), associated with rearrangement of the *bcl*-2 oncogene and characteristic of follicular lymphoma.

iv. The CT scan shows a high-density lesion of the hypothalamic region, and this was presumably responsible for her disorder of temperature control and her sleep disorder.

The lesion was not amenable to biopsy but her symptoms responded to local radiotherapy. It is likely that the low-grade tumour had transformed into a high-grade neoplasm. A fungal infection or some other infective process could cause a similar picture. This particular patient also had retroperitoneal lymphadenopathy and subsequently developed renal failure. Her central nervous system lymphoma recurred, and she presented with visual disturbance. A repeat CT scan (**26e**) showed a lesion affecting her occipital cortex. Subsequent lymph node biopsies (**26f**) showed that her histology had progressed from predominantly small cell to mixed centrocytic–centroblastic and finally to large cell (centroblastic, high-grade) lymphoma (**26g**).

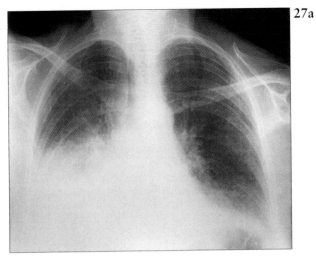

27a

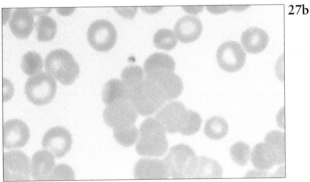

27b

27 A 53-year-old woman, who is a heavy smoker, develops a productive cough and receives oral amoxycillin. Her symptoms persist and 1 week later she develops progressive tiredness and shortness of breath. Her full blood count shows:

Hb	8.7 g/dl
MCV	110 fl
WBC	11.3 x 10⁹/l (neutrophils 71%)
Platelets	305 x 10⁹/l

i. Comment on the chest X-ray (27a).
ii. Comment on the blood film (27b).
iii. What is the likely diagnosis?
iv. What further investigations are indicated?
v. How would you treat her?

27 i. The chest X-ray shows evidence of a lobar pneumonia affecting the right base.

ii. The blood film shows marked auto-agglutination, suggesting the presence of cold agglutinins.

iii. Auto-immune haemolytic anaemia with cold agglutinins secondary to *Mycoplasma pneumoniae* infection.

iv. A DAT test was positive, and demonstrated both IgM and complement on the red cell surface. Mycoplasma titres should be assessed.

The blood group should be determined and the cold agglutinin titre should be measured. Auto-immune haemolytic anaemia following *M. pneumoniae* infection is typically associated with an increased titre of anti-I antibodies, which react optimally at 4°C. Patients with cold reactive auto-antibodies often develop acrocyanosis and Raynaud's phenomenon, as the periphery is at a lower temperature than the body core. The suggested mechanism of auto-immune haemolytic anaemia following *M. pneumoniae* infection is that antibodies to the organism cross-react with the I antigen, which is normally expressed on all adult red cells. Other infections that may lead to auto-immune haemolytic anaemia include syphilis and infectious mononucleosis.

v. Treatment is with erythromycin.

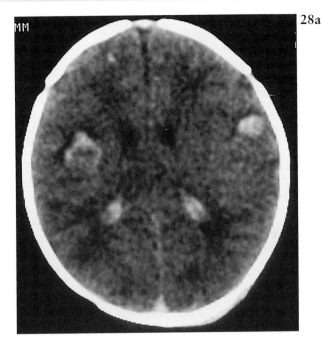
28a

28 A full-term neonate is found to have purpura, ecchymosis, and difficulty in breathing. A full blood count shows:

Hb 17.3 g/dl
WBC 16.4 x 10⁹/l
Platelets 4 x 10⁹/l

A CT scan was performed (**28a**). The mother has had one previous pregnancy 4 years ago, and there were no complications during the current pregnancy.

i. Comment on the appearance of the CT scan.
ii. What important causes would you consider for the thrombocytopenia?
iii. How should the child be treated?
iv. What advice would you give regarding future pregnancy?

28 i. The CT scan shows evidence of acute haemorrhage.

ii. Important causes of neonatal thrombocytopenia are genetic, congenital and acquired. Genetic causes are rare, but include thrombocytopenia with absent radii (TAR syndrome). Congenital infection (rubella, CMV, toxoplasmosis) should be excluded by serological tests on mother and culture studies of the neonate. Congenital immune thrombocytopenia may arise through transplacental passage of IgG antiplatelet antibodies in mothers with idiopathic thrombocytopenic purpura, or may present as neonatal alloimmune thrombocytopenia. Mothers who lack certain platelet antigens (most commonly PLA1, also called HPA-1a) will make antibodies if sensitised by previous pregnancy or transfusion. Acquired causes include sepsis, disseminated intravascular coagulation, and drugs.

iii. Maternal serum was found to contain anti-PLA1 antibodies. The mother's own platelets were PLA1 negative, and the father and both children were PLA1 positive (as are more than 95% of people). Thus, a diagnosis of neonatal alloimmune thrombocytopenia was made. The child received transfusion of PLA1-negative platelets, which were continued until the child was able to maintain an unsupported count of more than 50×10^9/l. This occurred within 3 weeks as the titre of transplacentally derived antibody fell. High-dose intravenous immunoglobulin may also help to elevate the neonatal platelet count.

iv. The partner should be tested and, if he is homozygous HPA-1a positive, as is likely, then future children will be affected. The fetal platelet count can be monitored during pregnancy and, if required, HPA-1a negative platelets can be transfused as prophylaxis against bleeding. Delivery should be by elective Caesarean section.

All blood components for intra-uterine transfusion should be irradiated to minimise the risk of graft versus host disease.

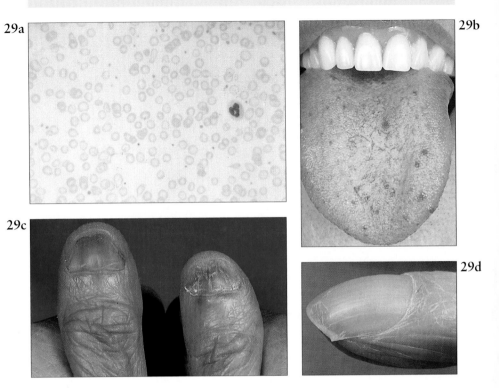

29 i. What abnormalities are shown in this blood film (**29a**)? What is the likely diagnosis?
ii. What abnormality is shown (**29b**)? What is the likely diagnosis?
iii. What abnormality is shown(**29c**)? What is the likely diagnosis?
iv. What abnormality is shown (**29d**)? What are the possible causes?

29e

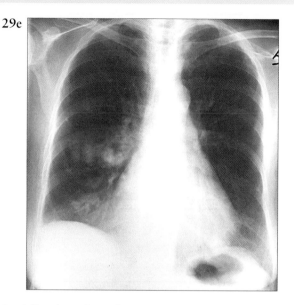

29 i. This blood film shows hypochromic, microcytic red blood cells with occasional target cells. The features suggest iron deficiency.

ii. This patient has multiple telangiectasia over the tongue and lips, and suffers from hereditary haemorrhagic telangiectasia (Osler–Weber–Rendu syndrome). Chronic iron deficiency may result from gastrointestinal blood loss. The condition is inherited as an autosomal dominant.

iii. The nail appearances are those of koilonychia (spoon-shaped nails), which is seen in chronic iron deficiency. Other skin and mucosal changes in iron deficiency include:

- Brittle nails.
- Angular cheilitis.
- Postcricoid and pharyngeal webs (Plummer–Vinson syndrome), which may present as dysphagia.

iv. Clubbing. This was associated with pulmonary arteriovenous fistulae in hereditary haemorrhagic telangiectasia, as shown in the chest X-ray (**29e**) Other causes of clubbing include:

- Carcinoma of the bronchus.
- Suppurative lung disease.
- Cyanotic congenital heart disease.
- Cirrhosis.
- Inflammatory bowel disease.

30 This patient gives a 3-month history of gradually increasing tiredness and lack of energy. Her blood count shows:

Hb	9.4 g/dl
MCV	100 fl
WBC	4.7 x 10⁹/l
Platelets	130 x 10⁹/l

i. What is the diagnosis (30a, 30b)?
ii. What other information should be sought in the history?
iii. What other haematological complications may occur?

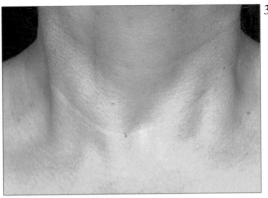
30a

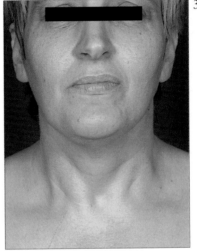
30b

30c 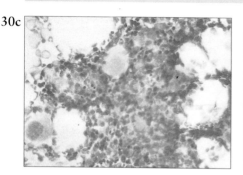 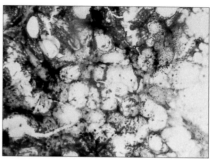 30d

30 i. This patient is suffering from hypothyroidism.
ii. This patient had a strong family history of thyroid disease. Voice changes, intolerance to cold, slow mentation, and shortness of breath arising through associated congestive cardiac failure (or, less commonly, pericardial effusion) are other frequent symptoms.
iii. Both hyperthyroidism and hypothyroidism are associated with mild anaemia, which is usually normochromic and normocytic, though there may be a macrocytosis in hypothyroidism.

Iron deficiency may arise through associated menorrhagia in hypothyroidism, and defective iron utilisation may occur as in the anaemia of chronic disease. There is an increased incidence of pernicious anaemia in patients with auto-immune hypothyroidism, as well as in those with hypoadrenalism, hypoparathyroidism, and diabetes mellitus. Mild normochromic normocytic anaemia may also occur in Addison's disease, hypopituitarism, and hypogonadism. Phaeochromocytoma is occasionally associated with erythrocytosis.

A neutrophil leukocytosis may occur in Cushing's syndrome and phaeochromocytoma, and diabetes mellitus is associated with impaired neutrophil function. Abnormal platelet function is reported in diabetes mellitus and hyperthyroidism, and hypercoagulability is of clinical significance in diabetes, following oestrogen therapy, and in Cushing's syndrome.

In the anaemia of chronic disease (ACD), the serum iron is low but the iron binding capacity is also low, whereas it is raised in iron deficiency. A low serum ferritin indicates iron deficiency, but ferritin may rise in inflammatory conditions. Assessment of iron status may therefore require bone marrow examination. 30c shows a Perl's stain with reduced iron stores. 30d shows normal/increased stores. In ACD, iron may be present in stores but absent in developing erythroblasts.

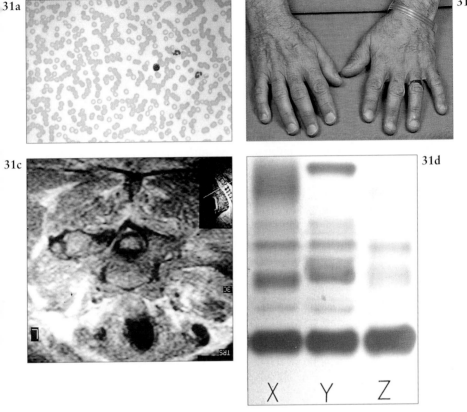

31 A 62-year-old man has progressive onset of pain at the back of the neck. He has also noted weakness of his hands over a 3-week period, and he is having difficulty grasping objects. He reports numbness along the inner aspect of his arm. Investigations show:

Hb	9.4 g/dl	Platelets	137 x 10⁹/l
MCV	87	ESR	110 mm/hour
WBC	7.4 x 10⁹/l		

Hb 9.4 g/dl — MCV 87 — WBC 7.4 x 10^9/l — Platelets 137 x 10^9/l — ESR 110 mm/hour

i.   Comment on the blood film (**31a**).
ii. Comment on the photograph of the patient's hands (**31b**).
iii. Comment on the CT scan of his neck (**31c**).
iv. Comment on the protein electrophoretic strip (**31d**):
• Lane *x* is from a patient with cirrhosis.
• Lane *y* is from the patient.
• Lane *z* is a normal control.
v.   What is the diagnosis?
vi. What further investigations are indicated?

31: Answers

31 i. The blood film shows rouleaux formation. This is frequently seen in association with a raised ESR and should raise suspicion of an underlying disorder of plasma proteins, eg, polyclonal or monoclonal increase in gamma globins.

ii. The hands show bilateral changes of muscle wasting, and are consistent with a T1 cord lesion.

iii. CT of the neck shows an extradural tumour affecting the cervical spine.

iv. Protein electrophoresis on the patient (lane *y*) shows a monoclonal band in the gammaglobulin region with a corresponding reduction in the other immunoglobulins. Lane *x* shows polyclonal hypergammaglobulinaemia. The paraprotein band is further characterised by immunofixation, and clearly reacts with only IgG and kappa antisera (31e).

v. Multiple myeloma.

vi. A full biochemical assessment is needed, including urea, calcium, liver function tests, creatinine clearance, immunoglobulins, paraprotein quantitation in serum and urine, including screening for Bence–Jones protein.

Bone marrow aspirate and possibly aspirate of the cervical lesion will confirm the diagnosis. A skeletal survey is more sensitive than a bone scan at detecting myeloma deposits. Both the b2 microglobulin level and the plasma C reactive protein give useful prognostic information in myeloma.

Myeloma cells are monoclonal B lymphocytes, and as such have a discrete rearrangement of their immunoglobulin genes. This rearrangement can be detected by the Southern blot technique (31f). Whereas granulocytes (G) have a germ-line configuration of their immunoglobulin genes, bone marrow (BM) and peripheral blood mononuclear cells (MN) have a population of cells with a discrete rearrangement. The detection of rearranged immunoglobulin genes is a powerful technique for characterising B cell malignancies, and offers a sensitive method for detecting minimal residual disease after chemotherapy.

POEMS syndrome is the association of polyneuropathy with organomegaly, endocrinopathy, a monoclonal gammopathy and skin lesions. The bone marrow aspirate (31g) shows an increase in plasma cells.

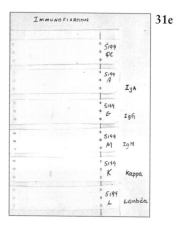

31e

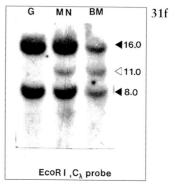

31f

EcoR I ,C$_\lambda$ probe

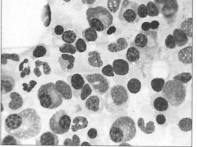

31g

32 A 9-year-old boy presents with a long history of anaemia. It was first noted when he was 4, at which time a blood count showed:

Hb   6.5 g/dl
MCV   56 fl
MCHC   29 g/dl

Since this initial presentation, he has received blood transfusions on 3 occasions. He has hepatosplenomegaly.

i. Comment on the blood film (**32a, 32b**). What is the likely diagnosis?

ii. Comment on the boy's facial appearance (**32c**).

iii. What is the pathogenesis of this condition?

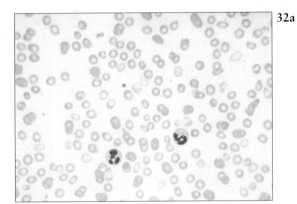

32a

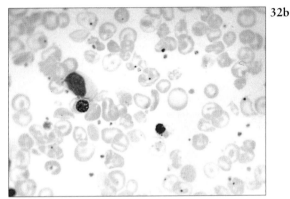

32b

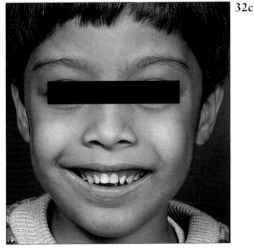

32c

32d
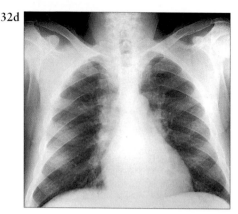

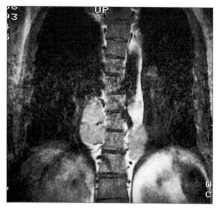
32e

COURTESY OF DR S J PAREKH

32 i. The blood film shows hypochromic microcytic red cells and occasional circulating nucleated red cells. The likely diagnosis is beta thalassaemia of a severity greater than thalassaemia trait but with an age of onset later than beta thalassaemia major. The patient is able to survive without regular transfusion therapy, suggesting he has beta thalassaemia intermedia.

ii. The facial appearance ('chipmunk face') confirms maxillary enlargement due to extramedullary haemopoiesis. Skeletal abnormalities are often prominent in thalassaemia intermedia as a result of chronic extramedullary haemopoiesis.

iii. The commonest mechanism of amelioration of beta thalassaemia major is co-inheritance of alpha thalassaemia. This is because excess deposition of alpha chains is an important cause of ineffective erythropoiesis and haemolysis in beta thalassaemia major; the extent of such deposition is lessened if the patient has defective formation of alpha chains by virtue of having alpha thalasseamia trait.

Some patients have additional genetic mutations that serve to increase gamma chain (and hence Hb F) production. Furthermore, although some beta gene mutations lead to complete absence of beta globin chain synthesis (βo), others are compatible with some degree of production. Thus, β+/β+ frequently produces a less severe phenotype than βo/βo.

Splenectomy may be of value, both in reducing splenic pooling of transfused red cells and in reducing haemolysis and extramedullary haemopoiesis. Skeletal abnormalities can be quite dramatic: a paraspinal mass is visible on the plain chest X-ray (32d), and extramedullary haemopoiesis in a paraspinal mass is shown on the MRI scan (32e).

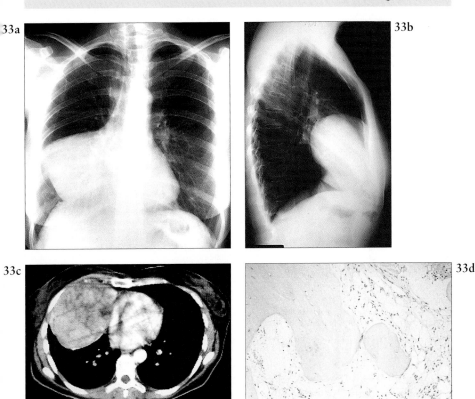

33 A 23-year-old woman gives a 3-month history of progressively increasing tiredness with bruising, malaise and menorrhagia. On examination she is anaemic and has multiple bruises. A full blood count shows:

Hb	6.9 g/dl
WBC	1.1 x 10⁹/l (neutrophils 0.3 x 10⁹/l)
Platelets	17 x 10⁹/l

Her chest X-ray (PA and lateral – 33a, 33b), thoracic CT scan (33c) and bone marrow trephine biopsy (33d) are illustrated.
i.   What abnormality is shown on the chest X-ray and CT scan?
ii. What abnormality is shown on the bone marrow trephine biopsy?
iii. What further investigations should be undertaken?
iv. What are the treatment options for this condition?

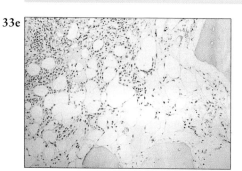 33e

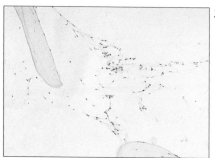 33f

33 i. The chest X-ray shows an abnormal mass in the anterior mediastinum which, notwithstanding the unusual appearance, turned out at surgery to be a thymoma.

ii. Her bone marrow trephine biopsy confirms that she has aplastic anaemia. The degree of cellularity is quite variable, not only in normals but also in patients with aplastic anaemia, and two additional trephine biopsies from aplastic patients (33e, 33f) demonstrate this.

iii. Thymoma may be associated with red cell aplasia and was presumably aetiologically related to marrow aplasia in this case. Other investigations that should be performed in aplastic anaemia:

- Antinuclear factor.
- Ham's test (to exclude coexistent paroxysmal nocturnal haemoglobinuria).
- Serology for hepatitis virus infection.
- Immunoglobulins (thymoma may be associated with hypogammaglobulinaemia).
- Co-culture of serum or T cells with patient's own marrow and normal marrow (this may demonstrate a serum or cellular inhibitor of haemopoiesis).

iv. This patient underwent thymectomy, though it should be emphasised that thymoma is only very rarely associated with aplastic anaemia and is more frequently associated with isolated red cell aplasia. Supportive care with red cells, platelets (filtered, to reduce the incidence of HLA sensitisation) and antibiotics and antifungal agents is valuable. Recombinant haemopoietic growth factors are of limited value in this condition, but antilymphocyte globulin, methylprednisolone and cyclosporin A are beneficial in over 50% of patients. A progestogen (eg, norethisterone) or the oral contraceptive pill is frequently helpful in controlling menorrhagia.

Allogeneic bone marrow transplantation from a histocompatible sibling, if available, should be considered in any patient under 50 with severe aplastic anaemia (platelets < 20 x 10^9/l, neutrophils < 0.5 x 10^9/l).

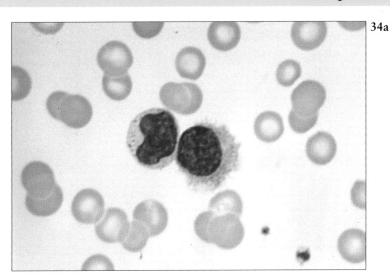

34a

34 A 62-year-old man is generally unwell and complaining of increased tiredness over a 3-month period. He has had 2 recent episodes of chest infection requiring antibiotic therapy. On examination he is pale. The tip of the spleen is palpable, but there is no jaundice and no lymphadenopathy. His full blood count shows:

Hb   9.1 g/dl
WBC   3.9 x 10⁹/l (lymphocytes 65%, neutrophils 32%)
Platelets   91 x 10⁹/l

A bone marrow aspirate is unsuccessful.

i. Comment on the blood film appearances (34a).
ii. What is the diagnosis?
iii. How would you confirm the diagnosis?
iv. How is this condition treated?

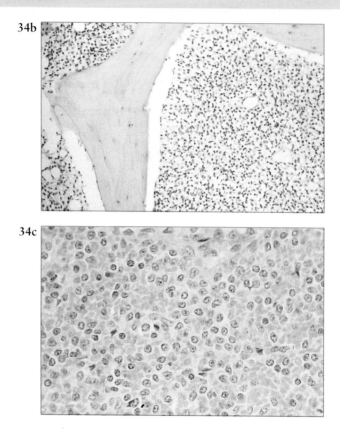

34b

34c

34   i. The blood film shows abnormal circulating lymphoid cells with cytoplasmic projections.

ii. The morphology of the circulating cells, history of pancytopenia and splenomegaly and an unsuccessful aspirate strongly suggest hairy cell leukaemia.

iii. A marrow trephine biopsy (34b) will often show a characteristic appearance of large cells with plentiful cytoplasm. The acid phosphatase reaction is usually positive and tartrate resistant (TRAP). Immunophenotypic analysis of the lymphocytes will show them to be monoclonal B cells and CD11c positive (T hairy cell leukaemia is exceedingly rare).

iv. A number of treatments are available in addition to supportive care. Effective chemotherapeutic agents include 2-chlorodeoxyadenosine, deoxycoformycin and interferon, while splenectomy has an important role in those patients who have good marrow function. Splenic infiltration by hairy cells is shown in 34c.

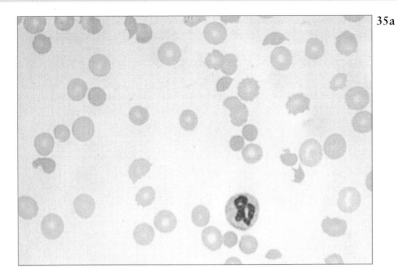
35a

35 A 27-year-old pregnant woman (36 weeks) becomes acutely unwell with fever, purpuric lesions over her limbs, and declining consciousness. A full blood count shows:

Hb	7.5 g/dl
MCV	110 fl
Reticulocytes	12%
WBC	26.4 x 10⁹/l (neutrophils 86%)
Platelets	14 x 10⁹/l
Urea	67 mmol/l

i. Comment on the blood film (35a).
ii. What is the differential diagnosis, and what further investigations are required?
iii. What treatment would you recommend?

35b

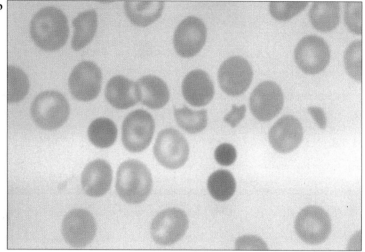

35 i. The blood film shows red cell fragmentation, polychromasia, spherocytes, thrombocytopenia and target cells.

ii. The association of fever, fragmentation haemolysis, renal failure, neurological changes and thrombocytopenia suggests thrombotic thrombocytopenic purpura (TTP), which has an increased frequency in pregnancy. It must be distinguished from disseminated intravascular coagulation (eg, in association with sepsis, amniotic fluid embolism, antepartum haemorrhage, and retention of a dead fetus or products of conception), and a coagulation screen is required urgently. This was normal in this case. Liver function tests were normal, differentiating this from HELLP (haemolytic anaemia, elevated liver enzymes and low platelets) syndrome and acute fatty liver of pregnancy (35b shows target cells due to coexistent liver disease in a case of TTP). A buccal biopsy may be helpful and may show evidence of microvascular thrombosis. Infusion of fresh frozen plasma (FFP), or plasma exchange with FFP, is advised. Platelet transfusion should be avoided, as it may aggravate thrombosis. Prostacyclin infusion, steroid therapy, anti-platelet drugs and splenectomy are not of proven benefit.

iii. Urgent obstetric and haematological review is required, but unlike the situation in disseminated intravascular coagulation, there is no immediate indication to deliver the fetus; indeed, it may be safer to delay this until the mother's condition has been stabilised.

36 A 47-year-old man of Greek–Cypriot origin was noticed to have a hypochromic microcytic anaemia at an insurance medical examination. He was commenced on iron replacement therapy, and this has been continued since, but now, 6 months later, his blood count is unchanged:

Hb	9.6 g/dl
MCV	62 fl
MCHC	29 g/dl

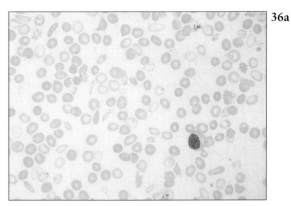

36a

On examination, he has a palpable spleen.

i. Comment on the blood film (**36a**).
ii. What preparation has been made (**36b**)?
iii. Comment on the haemoglobin electrophoresis result (**36c**: Y is the patient, Z is an A/S control, and X is a normal control).
iv. What is the likely diagnosis? What is the pathogenesis of this condition?

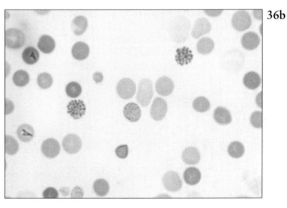

36b

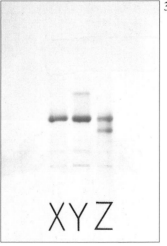

36c

36 i. The blood film shows hypochromic microcytic changes consistent with a thalassaemic disorder. Iron deficiency in a man this age should immediately prompt a search for a cause, eg, gastrointestinal blood loss, and iron replacement therapy should not be commenced until iron deficiency is proven (eg, by estimation of serum ferritin).

ii. This is a 'haemoglobin H' preparation. It shows the characteristic 'golf ball' appearance of red cells, indicating haemoglobin H disease. The inclusions are precipitates of Hb H (B_4, tetramers of beta chains).

iii. There is a fast-migrating band, which is haemoglobin H (tetramers of beta chains).

iv. Haemoglobin H disease. Each normal individual has 4 alpha genes, 2 on each chromosome 16. Alpha thalassaemia is an autosomal recessive disorder. Absence of alpha globin chain production usually arises through deletion of the corresponding gene. Individuals who have no alpha globin genes have alpha thalassaemia major (--/--), and cannot even make fetal haemoglobin (Hb F,$\alpha_2\gamma_2$). They present as hydrops foetalis and late fetal intrauterine death at 30–34 weeks' gestation. At the other extreme, individuals with 2 or 3 functional alpha globin genes (-α/$\alpha\alpha$, α-/α-, or $\alpha\alpha$/--) are completely asymptomatic and will typically have a normal Hb and a degree of microcytosis. Haemoglobin H disease arises through loss of 3 alpha globin genes (α-/--). It is a very mild haemoglobinopathy and it typically does not require any therapy other than folic acid supplementation.

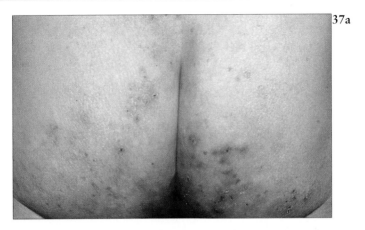
37a

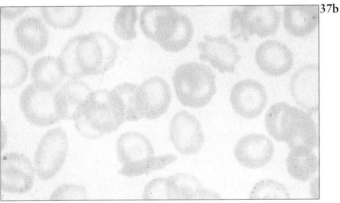
37b

37 A 24-year-old female develops a pruritic rash over her flexor surfaces, at the nape of her back and over her buttocks (37a). The rash is localised, vesicular, and intensely pruritic. She has also noted fatigue, weight loss of 3 kg over the preceding 2 months, and occasional bouts of central abdominal pain. Her bowels are loose. A full blood count shows:

Hb	9.1 g/dl
MCV	103 fl
WBC	3.6 x 10⁹/l
Platelets	110 x 10⁹/l

i. What is the dermatological diagnosis?
ii. What abnormalities are seen on the blood film (37b)?
iii. What further investigations are required?

37c

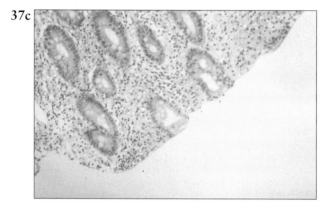

37d

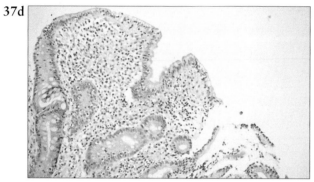

37 i. Dermatitis herpetiformis. Dapsone is the customary therapy, which at high doses can lead to oxidant damage and haemolytic anaemia even in normal individuals.

ii. The blood film shows occasional macrocytes, irregularly contracted red cells, target cells, and Howell–Jolly bodies. These features suggest hyposplenism.

iii. She probably has coeliac disease complicated by dermatitis herpetiformis, hyposplenism, and folic acid deficiency secondary to malabsorption.

Her serum and red cell folate levels, calcium, albumin, vitamin D and parathormone level should be estimated. She also requires a jejunal or duodenal biopsy to confirm the diagnosis. A duodenal biopsy in coeliac disease (**37c, 37d**) may show subtotal villous atrophy, crypt hyperplasia, and inflammatory cells in the lamina propria.

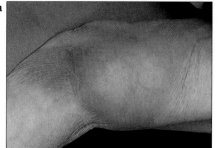
38a

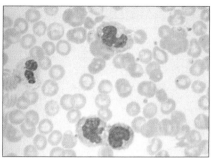
38b

38 A 52-year-old man is found to have an abnormal blood count during the course of routine investigation. He is in good health with no symptoms. He does not have bruising and has never suffered excessive bleeding following previous surgery. There is no family history of excessive bleeding. On examination he is found to have a markedly enlarged spleen. Investigations show:

Hb	13.4g/dl
WBC	51.3 x 10⁹/l
Platelets	147 x 10⁹/l
Liver function tests	normal
Protein electrophoresis	normal
PT	12 seconds (control 11–13 seconds)
APTT	74 seconds (control 30–40 seconds)
APTT after 50:50 mix with normal plasma	45 seconds
Factor VIII level	74% (normal range 50 –150%)
Factor IX level	86% (normal range 50 –150%)
Ivy template bleeding time	5 minutes (control up to 9 minutes)

A splenectomy is performed uneventfully after appropriate further investigation and treatment of his coagulation disorder.

Two months later, he trips while walking and injures his left arm (38a). His blood film is illustrated (38b).

i. What is the likely cause of the elevated white cell count with splenomegaly?
ii. What is the likely cause of his abnormal coagulation?
iii. How are these conditions treated?

38c

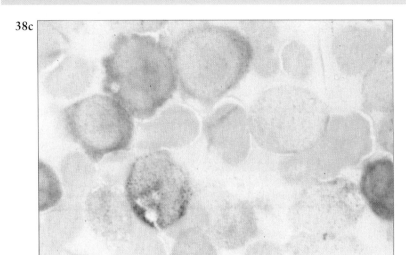

38 i. He has chronic myelomonocytic leukemia (CMML). This is a form of myelodysplasia and abnormal granulocytes accompany increased numbers of mature monocytes. Splenomegaly is usually present. It is unusual to present below the age of 60. A butyrate esterase stain shows these cells to be positive (38c).

ii. The isolated prolonged APTT, which corrects well when normal plasma is added, suggests a defect in the intrinsic pathway. Mixing experiments can also be done with aged plasma and plasma which has been absorbed with aluminium hydroxide gel; the former is deficient in factors V and VIII:C, while the latter is deficient in factors II, VII, IX and X. Both of these preparations would correct the abnormality observed in this patient, which was due to inherited factor XI deficiency. This is an autosomal recessive condition associated with a mild bleeding tendency; it occurs at high frequency in Ashkenazi Jews (approximately 10% are heterozygous carriers). Heterogeneous molecular abnormalities have been identified. Deficiencies of Factor XII, prekallikrein and high molecular weight kininogen can all lead to an isolated prolonged APTT but are usually clinically silent.

iii. Chronic myelomonocytic leukemia is a slowly progressive condition which is usually treated with oral chemotherapy (eg, hydroxyurea or etoposide). Splenectomy is helpful if patients become transfusion-dependent or if there are symptoms due to an enlarged organ. Transformation to acute leukemia occurs with a median interval of 18–24 months, but intensive chemotherapy is rarely successful. Younger patients should be considered for intensive therapy, possibly followed by bone marrow transplantation; however, this particular patient did not have a suitable donor.

Factor XI deficiency is best treated with purified Factor XI concentrate. The two conditions occurred together in this patient by coincidence.

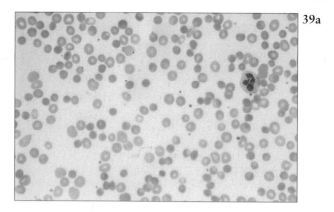

39a

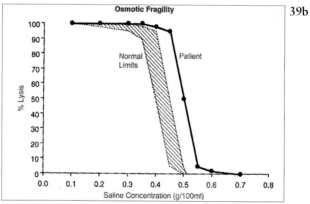

39b

39 A 17-year-old male has been noted to be jaundiced on several occasions. He him-self feels completely well. On examination he is slightly jaundiced. There are no signs of chronic liver disease, but the tip of the spleen is palpable. Investigations show:

Hb	13.4 g/dl
MCV	85 fl
WBC	7.6 x 10⁹/l (differential normal)
Platelets	185 x 10⁹/l
Reticulocytes	8%
DAT test	negative

i. Comment on the blood film (39a).
ii. Comment on the results of the osmotic fragility test (39b).
iii. What is the diagnosis?
iv. How should he be treated?

39c

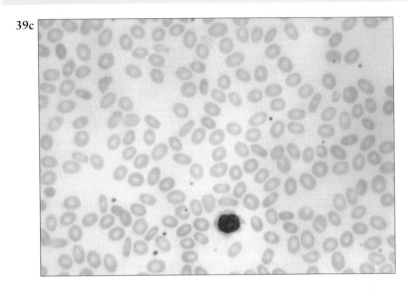

39 i. The blood film shows polychromasia with spherocytes.

ii. The graph of his osmotic fragility test shows his red cells to be abnormally suscep-tible to lysis in hypo-osmolar solution, in comparison with a normal control. This tendency is exaggerated by incubation of his red cells for 24 hours.

iii. With a negative direct antiglobulin test excluding auto-immune haemolytic anaemia, the likeliest diagnosis is hereditary spherocytosis. This is due to an inherited (autosomal dominant) defect in red cell membrane proteins. Hereditary elliptocytosis (**39c**) is not usually associated with haemolysis.

iv. He should receive folic acid supplements.

Splenectomy (preceded by pneumococcal and *Haemophilus influenzae* B vaccine and followed by long-term prophylaxis with penicillin V) is curative, but recom-mended only in symptomatic patients or in those with recurrent biliary problems due to pigment gallstones. Parvovirus infection can lead to aplastic crisis.

40 A 31-year-old male gives a 2- to 3-week history of fever, bruising and tiredness. There is no palpable splenomegaly. A full blood count shows:

Hb   6.7 g/dl
WBC   1.3 x 10⁹/l
 (blasts 12%,
  neutrophils 61%)
Platelets   12 x 10⁹/l

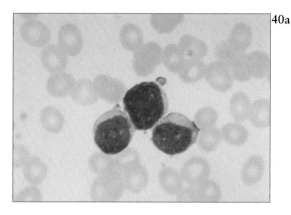

Bone marrow aspiration is unsuccessful, and a trephine biopsy is performed.

i. Comment on the blood film appearances (**40a**).

ii. Comment on the bone marrow trephine appearances (**40b**). What does the reticulin stain (**40c**) show?

iii. Which further tests may help in making a diagnosis?

iv. What is the likely diagnosis?

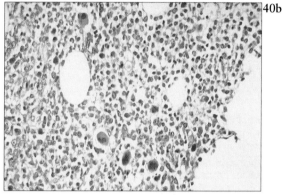

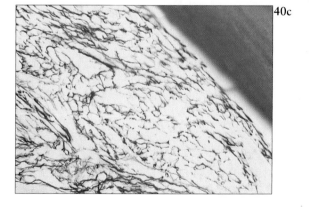

40 i. The blood film shows occasional circulating blasts, presumably leukaemic.

ii. The trephine biopsy shows increased numbers of megakaryocytes and scattered foci of immature blasts. The reticulin stains shows increased reticulin fibres, indicating a degree of marrow fibrosis. This fibrosis explains the failure to obtain an aspirate.

iii. A full clinical and radiological assessment should be undertaken. The absence of splenomegaly and virtually normal red cell morphology makes chronic myelofibrosis (which is in any event very rare at this age) unlikely. The picture is one of acute myelofibrosis, and further attempts should be made to concentrate and characterise the blast cells. This may best be done from peripheral blood. Cytochemistry and immunocytochemistry using monoclonal antibodies are powerful additional techniques. Myeloid blasts are usually Sudan Black positive (**40d**), whereas blasts in myelomonocytic leukaemias show positivity for chloroacetate (blue) and butyrate (brown) esterase (**40e**). Erythroid blasts are usually positive for glycophorin A.

A positive platelet peroxidase reaction, visualised by electron microscopy, and monoclonal antibody reactivity with anti-glycoprotein IIB/IIIA antibodies are features of megakaryoblastic leukaemia. Light microscopy of the initial Romanovsky stain may show Auer rods (**40f**), which is pathognomic of AML. The M4 Eo variant of AML of the M4 (myelomonocytic) type (**40g**) is characterised by abnormal eosinophils, and is usually associated with the presence of inversion of chromosome 16.

iv. The diagnosis in this case of acute onset of myelofibrosis was acute megakaryoblastic leukaemia (AML M7). Other possibilities are myelodysplasia, marrow infiltration by secondary carcinoma or lymphoma, and rarely a non-malignant disorder such as systemic lupus erythematosus.

41 A 12-year-old boy has a long history of regular red cell transfusions. These began when he was 1 year old. At that time, he had presented with a blood count:

Hb   3.1 g/dl
MCV   52 fl

His blood film is shown (**41a, 41b**).
i. What is the diagnosis?
ii. What is the pathogenesis?
iii. What abnormality is illustrated by the skull X-ray (**41c**)?
iv. What are the principles of management of this condition?

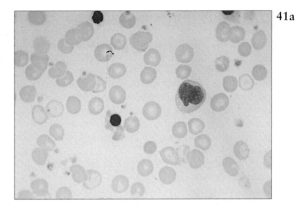
41a

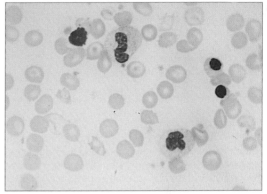
41b

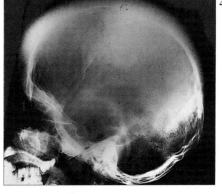
41c

41 i. Beta thalassemia major. There are target cells, hypochromic, microcytic cells, and circulating nucleated red cells.

ii. Beta thalassemia major arises through partial or complete failure of synthesis of beta globin chains, and thus causes impaired haemoglobin synthesis and chronic anaemia. Inheritance is as an autosomal recessive condition. The defect in the beta globin gene (situated alongside the gamma and delta genes on chromosome 11) is usually a point mutation affecting expression of the gene or processing of the messenger RNA. A diverse range of mutations is recorded, and this diversity is a cause of the variability in the clinical severity of the condition.

iii. The skull X-ray shows a 'hair-on-end' appearance, which is due to extramedullary haemopoiesis.

iv. The cornerstone of current management is long-term transfusion therapy. A red cell transfusion is required every 3–5 weeks, and attempts should be made to minimise sensitisation to red cell antigens (by use of genotyped cells) and HLA antigens (by use of filtered blood). Splenectomy may be beneficial, but is best delayed until after the age of 5 to reduce the risk of postsplenectomy infection.

A consequence of transfusion therapy is iron overload. Iron deposition in tissues leads to diverse clinical effects on many organs:

- Skin (pigmentation).
- Heart (cardiomyopathy).
- Liver (cirrhosis).
- Endocrine organs and pancreas (diabetes mellitus, growth impairment, delayed puberty).

Iron chelation therapy is usually administered in the form of parenteral desferrioxamine (typically given by subcutaneous infusion over 12 hours, 5 nights each week, with oral vitamin C), though orally active agents are now on clinical trial. Bone marrow transplantation is curative for selected patients.

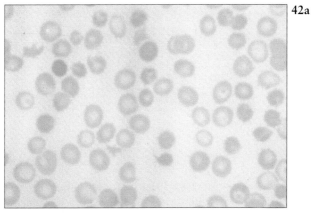

42a

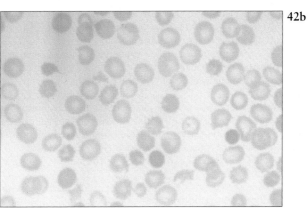

42b

42 A 36-year-old man is referred for investigation of thrombocytopenia. He has recently developed jaundice, tiredness and lack of libido. A blood count shows:

Hb	9.3 g/dl
WBC	3.1 x 10⁹/l
Platelets	78 x 10⁹ /l

Hb   9.3 g/dl
WBC   3.1 x 10⁹/l
Platelets   78 x 10⁹ /l

The coagulation screen shows:

PT   18 seconds (NR 11–15)
PTTK   46 seconds (NR 30–40)

i. What abnormalities are shown in the blood film (**42a, 42b**)?
ii. What additional information should be sought in the history and clinical examination?
iii. What other haematological complications may occur?

42c
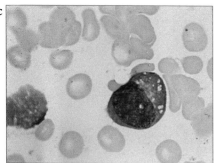

42d
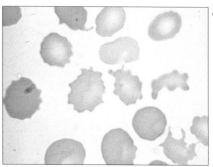

42 i. The blood film shows target cells, macrocytosis, occasional acanthocytes and thrombocytopenia. These findings, together with the presence of jaundice and the abnormal coagulation profile, suggest underlying chronic liver disease.
ii. This patient gave a history of travel to the Far East and an attack of hepatitis 5 years previously. He was found to have serological evidence of past infection with hepatitis A and C viruses. He had also been an intravenous drug abuser, and drank alcohol excessively. Examination revealed spider naevi, gynaecomastia, ascites, jaundice and splenomegaly. The probable cause of his pancytopenia is splenomegaly.
iii. Haematological complications of liver disease include:

• Anaemia – due to increased risk of gastrointestinal bleeding, dilution through increased plasma volume, sequestration within an enlarged spleen, abnormal erythropoietin metabolism, and haemolysis arising from alterations in red cell membrane lipids.
• Leukopenia – due to splenomegaly, paraproteinaemia in cirrhosis.
• Thrombocytopenia – due to splenomegaly, auto-immune destruction associated with chronic active hepatitis.
• Pancytopenia – associated with a hypercellular bone marrow in splenomegaly or aplastic anaemia (hypocellular bone marrow occurs in viral hepatitis).
• Coagulation changes – principally reduced production of coagulation factors (including factors II, VII, IX and X because of impaired absorption and activation of vitamin K), hypofibrinogenaemia and dysfibrinogenaemia, impaired clearance of activated coagulation factors, impaired production of inhibitors and regulators of coagulation and fibrinolysis (including anti-thrombin III, proteins C and S, and plasminogen) and impaired platelet function. Thus, these patients are at increased risk of developing thrombosis, haemorrhage and disseminated intravascular coagulation.
• Treatment-related haematological side-effects – eg, transfusion-associated viral infection.

Alcohol ingestion is a common cause of macrocytosis, thrombocytopenia and sideroblastic anaemia. 42c shows vacuolated erythroblasts in the marrow aspirate of a patient with alcohol related anaemia. Acanthocytosis (42d) also occurs in abetalipoproteinaemia.

43 A 9-year-old boy presents with a long-standing history of anaemia, renal impairment, growth retardation and skeletal deformity. A full blood count shows:

Hb	9.1 g/dl
MCV	103 fl
WBC	2.1 x 10⁹/l
(neutrophils 47%)	
Platelets	90 x 10⁹/l

A clinical photograph (**43a**), an X-ray (**43b**) of his hands and a bone marrow trephine biopsy (**43c**) are shown.

i. What is the diagnosis?
ii. What further tests are indicated to confirm the diagnosis?
iii. What other conditions may cause this haematological picture?
iv. How would you treat him?

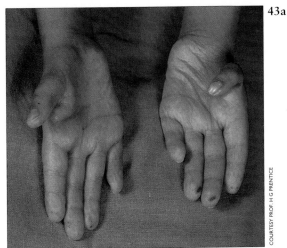

43a

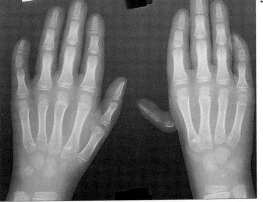

43b

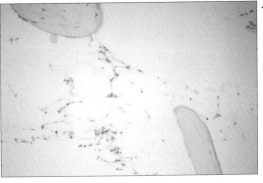

43c

43 i. Fanconi's anaemia. This is an autosomal recessive condition in which increased DNA fragility leads to multiple random chromosomal breaks; this in turn leads to aplastic anaemia. The trephine biopsy show hypocellularity of the marrow. Multiple skeletal changes may occur, such as hypoplasia of the thumb, the development of abnormal metacarpal bones and an incurved little finger, and absent radii. There can also be structural anomalies of the renal tract. Figure **43d** shows a patient with Fanconi's anaemia who has absent radii.

ii. The diagnosis is confirmed by cytogenetic (chromosome) analysis of stimulated cultures of haemopoietic cells from the bone marrow. An IVU should also be undertaken.

iii. Aplastic anaemia may occur secondary to drugs (chloramphenicol, sulphonamides, phenylbutazone and other non-steroidal anti-inflammatory drugs, gold, antithyroid drugs, tetracyclines, tricylic antidepressants, chlorpromazine) and toxins and chemicals (eg, benzene).

Reversible myelosuppression is inevitably associated with chemotherapy and radiotherapy. Certain viral infections (principally hepatitis, both A and B as well as non-A, non-B and, usually, non-C) are occasionally complicated by aplasia. Approximately 50% of cases are idiopathic, and immune mechanisms may operate.

Other congenital causes of bone marrow failure include ataxia telangiectasia and Bloom's syndrome, which, like Fanconi's anaemia, are associated with defects in DNA repair. They also have an increased risk of leukaemia as well as aplastic anaemia. Schwachmann's syndrome is an association of aplastic anaemia with exocrine pancreatic dysfunction.

iv. He requires assessment by a pediatrician, renal physician and endocrinologist. Androgen supplements may help to promote growth, and he may need treatment for renal impairment. Genetic counselling should be offered, as this is an autosomal recessive condition. The pancytopenia is mild and may respond to oral oxymetholone. Surgery (eg, dental therapy) will need to be covered by platelet transfusion, and infections will require antibiotic therapy. Definitive treatment (eg, bone marrow transplant) is only indicated if the counts deteriorate. These patients are at increased risk of malignancy, especially AML.

43d

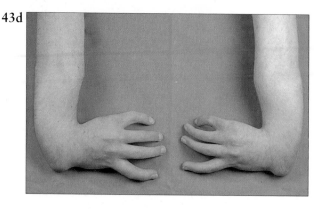

44 A 67-year-old female has bone pain affecting her spine and limbs. Two years ago she suffered a fracture of her lower femur, which has failed to heal properly. She complains of easy bruising and on examination has splenomegaly. Investigations show:

Hb	10.1 g/dl
MCV	82 fl
WBC	3.4 x 10⁹/l
(differential normal)	
Platelets	110 x 10⁹/l

i. What abnormalities are shown in the X-ray (**44a**) of her femur?
ii. What diagnosis is revealed by the bone marrow aspirate (**44b**) and trephine biopsy (**44c**)?
iii. How should she be treated?

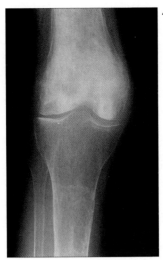

44a

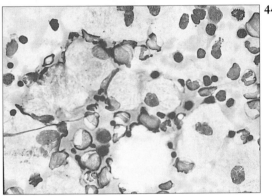

44b

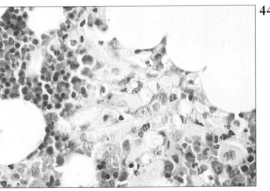

44c

44d

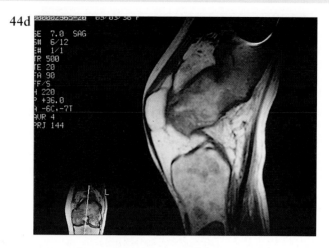

44 i. The X-ray shows loss of bony texture, and the MRI (44d) demonstrates replacement of the medullary cavity by abnormal tissue with multiple infarcts. The femoral appearances are those of the Erlenmeyer flask deformity of Gaucher's disease.

ii. Bone marrow aspirate and trephine biopsy show macrophages laden with lipids – typical Gaucher cells – suggesting she is suffering from Gaucher's disease of the chronic adult type (Type I). Type II and III Gaucher's disease also affect the central nervous system. Type I Gaucher's disease is due to mutations within glucocerebrosidase gene, which causes a deficiency of lysosomal beta glucocerebrosidase. This in turn leads to accumulation of glucocerebroside in reticuloendothelial cells.

iii. Although splenectomy may lead to haematological improvement, it can also lead to increased deposition of cerebroside in other tissues such as the skeleton.

Enzyme replacement therapy with glucocerebrosidase purified from human placenta is a promising new form of therapy. Allogeneic bone marrow transplantation has been performed successfully in young patients.

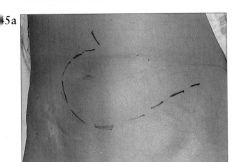

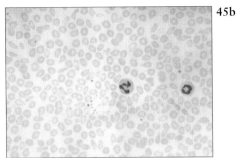

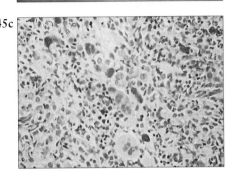

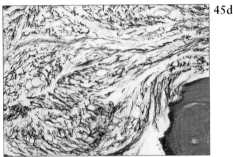

45 A 66-year-old woman has a 4-week history of gradually increasing tiredness. Examination reveals a markedly enlarged spleen, palpable 12 cm below the left costal margin (45a). Investigations show:

Hb	9.6 g/dl
MCV	81 fl
WBC	4.1 x 10⁹/l (differential normal)
Platelets	161 x 10⁹/l

Hb   9.6 g/dl
MCV   81 fl
WBC 4.1×10^9/l (differential normal)
Platelets 161 x 10^9/l

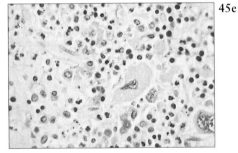

i. Comment on the blood film (45b).
ii. Comment on the haematoxylin and eosin (45c) and reticulin (45d) stains of the bone marrow trephine biopsy.
iii. A splenectomy is performed 1 year later. Comment on the spleen histology (45e).
iv. What is the diagnosis?
v. How is this condition generally treated?

45f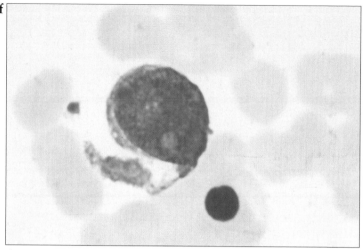

45 i. The blood film shows marked anisocytosis and poikilocytosis with macrocytes and occasional tear drop forms.
ii. Bone marrow reticulin is increased, indicating marrow fibrosis.
iii. Megakaryocytes, granulocytic cells, and erythroid cells are seen, indicating extramedullary haemopoiesis.
iv. Chronic idiopathic myelofibrosis.
v. Treatment is unsatisfactory. The marrow fibrosis is a reactive phenomenon, and the precise cause of increased fibrosis in this (and other) myeloproliferative disorders is unknown. A proportion of patients with myelofibrosis have a preceding history of polycythaemia rubra vera. Oral chemotherapy (eg, hydroxyurea) usually does not reduce fibrosis, but it can lead to a reduction in splenic size and will control the white cell count when the disease is in the proliferative phase. Folic acid is frequently helpful.

Supportive care, with red cell transfusions and occasionally platelet transfusions, is usually required. Splenectomy is usually needed at some point, as progressive splenomegaly contributes to an increasing transfusion requirement. Splenectomy should be preceded by pneumococcal and *Haemophilus influenzae* type B (Hib) vaccinations, and long-term penicillin prophylaxis is required after splenectomy. Splenic radiotherapy is worth trying in patients who are unfit for splenectomy. Transformation to acute leukaemia (often with a population of megakaryoblasts, 45f), occurs in the terminal stages.

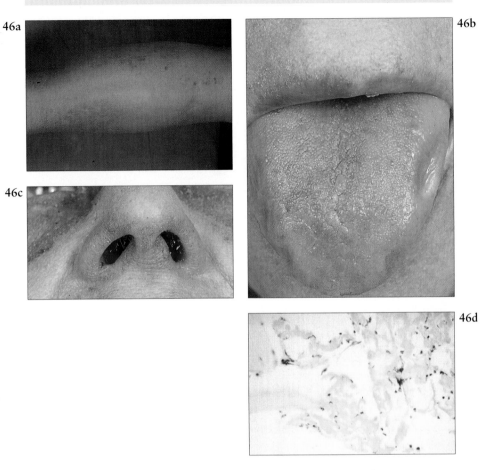

46 A 65-year-old woman presented for investigation of easy bruising (46a). Investigations showed:

Hb	9.5 g/dl
MCV	81 fl
WBC	9.2 x 10⁹/l
Platelets	137 x 10⁹/l
PT	12 seconds (control 11–13.5 seconds)
APTT	38 seconds (control 30–40 seconds)
Ivy template bleeding time	10.5 minutes (control 2–10 minutes)

i. Comment on the facial appearance (46b, 46c).
ii. Comment on the bone marrow trephine biopsy (46d).
iii. What is the diagnosis?
iv. What further investigations are required?

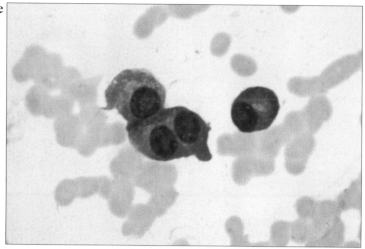

46e

46 i. She has abnormal skin infiltration around the nose and eyes, and an enlarged tongue. The history of excessive bruising with inconclusive coagulation profile (marginally prolonged bleeding time) suggests a disorder of skin or connective tissue, eg, amyloidosis.

ii. The bone marrow shows amyloidosis – homogenous pink-staining material (haematoxylin and eosin stain) or red-staining material (Congo red stain), which is birefringent to polarised light.

iii. Systemic amyloidosis. A skin biopsy will confirm this, and blood tests should be undertaken to characterise amyloid proteins. Amyloid light chains (AL) are seen in association with paraproteins and in primary amyloid, whereas protein A derived from serum amyloid-A (SAA) is seen in amyloidosis reactive to a systemic disease (eg, rheumatoid arthritis, chronic suppurative infection).

iv. A cause for the amyloid should be established (see above). In this patient, the amyloid was of AL type and she was found to suffer from myeloma. Other organs frequently involved in this form of amyloid include the heart, kidneys, liver, spleen, and nerves.

Reactive systemic amyloidosis typically affects the liver, spleen, kidneys, and marrow, but not usually the skin, tongue, heart, or nervous system.

An excess number of plasma cells is frequently present in the marrow aspirate (46e) and this patient was treated with chemotherapy as for multiple myeloma. She responded poorly to melphalan and prednisolone.

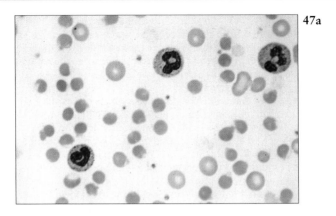

47a

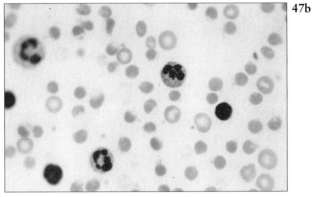

47b

47 A 7-year-old boy of Greek parents gives a 4-day history of fever, sore throat and abdominal pain. He has passed dark urine. He has been taking amoxycillin suspension for 2 days. There is no relevant family history and he has had no similar attacks previously, though his mother reveals that he did have prolonged neonatal jaundice. On examination he is clinically jaundiced and anaemic. Liver and spleen are not palpable. A full blood count shows:

Hb   6.1 g/dl
MCV   110 fl
WBC   17.3 x 10⁹/l (lymphocytes 46%, neutrophils 52%)
Platelets   307 x 10⁹/l
Reticulocytes are raised at 18%

i.   What is the diagnosis and how would you confirm it (blood film, 47a, 47b)?
ii. What precipitants are recognised?
iii. How would you manage this patient?
iv. What complications occur in the neonatal period in this condition?

97

47 i. The blood film shows polychromasia, anisocytosis and 'bite' cells, in which haemoglobin is separated from the red cell membrane.

ii. Acute haemolysis in an individual with glucose-6-phosphate dehydrogenase (G6PD) deficiency. G6PD deficiency is X-linked, and is the commonest inherited disease, with wide prevalence in Africa, Asia, the Middle East, and around the Mediterranean. Confirmation is by red cell enzyme assay or by performing a fluorescent screening test that detects NADPH production. G6PD is the first enzyme in the hexose monophosphate pathway, and it generates NADPH as an important source of reducing power for the red cell. G6PD deficiency renders the red cell susceptible to oxidant stress. Infection (probably viral, as evidenced by the lymphocytosis) is the likely precipitating factor in this case, but other precipitants would be the neonatal period, drugs (not amoxycillin, but principally sulphonamides, antimalarials, nalidixic acid and nitrofurantoin), and ingestion of fava beans (broad beans).

iii. He requires supportive management with encouragement of oral fluid intake, intravenous fluids and transfusion of packed red cells. Once the diagnosis is confirmed, he should receive a card informing which drugs and precipitants to avoid. He should also receive oral folic acid 5 mg/day, though haemolysis is usually only intermittent and is frequently very well compensated. Family studies will show his mother to be a carrier, and 50% of his male siblings are likely to be affected.

iv. Neonatal jaundice. G6PD deficiency is the commonest red cell enzymopathy to cause neonatal haemolysis and jaundice. Neonatal erythrocytes have an increased susceptibility to oxidative haemolysis (since they may have reduced concentrations of glutathione reductase, catalase and vitamin E) and this, combined with hepatic immaturity and G6PD deficiency within hepatocytes, predisposes to jaundice. This usually apears in the first to fourth day of life and unconjugated hyperbilirubinaemia may even lead to kernicterus. Phototherapy and exchange transfusion may be required.

The vast majority of individuals with G6PD deficiency suffer no symptoms unless challenged. Some 350 variant forms of the enzyme have been described, resulting from as many (usually single base) mutations within the gene. Individuals – especially heterozygous females – enjoy a degree of protection against *P. falciparium* malaria, as do heterozygotes (but emphatically not homozygous individuals) for sickle cell anaemia and thalassaemia.

48 A 17-year-old female has severe nose bleeds which have been intermittent over the past 3 years. She has had heavy periods ever since their onset at the age of 12. She is on oral iron therapy. She has never had surgery, but her grandmother died of bleeding after appendicectomy. On examination she is pale but otherwise normal. Investigations show:

Hb	9.6 g/dl
MCV	72 fl
WBC	9.3 x 10⁹/l
Platelets	163 x 10⁹/l

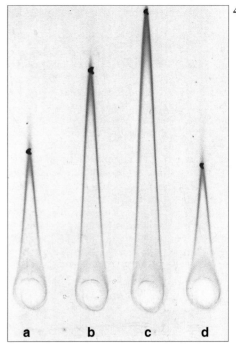

48a

Coagulation tests show:

PT	12 seconds (control 11–13 seconds)
PTTK	66 seconds (control 30–40 seconds)
Thrombin time	18 seconds (control 18–20 seconds)
PTTK with 50:50 mix of normal plasma	42 seconds (control 30–40 seconds)
Ivy template bleeding time	17 minutes (NR 5–10 minutes)

i. What abnormality is seen in the immunoprecipitation assay for Factor VIII-related antigen that was performed (48a)?
• Lanes *a*, *b*, and *c* are control plasma at concentrations of 12.5%, 25%, and 50%
• Lane *d* is neat patient plasma.
ii. What abnormality of platelet function typically occurs in this condition ?
iii. How is the condition treated?

48 i. This is an illustration of Laurel rocket electrophoresis. It demonstrates that the patient has a reduced level of Factor VIII-related antigen (VIII RAG). Normal range is 50–150%, and her level is approximately 10%.

ii. Defective aggregation with ristocetin.

iii. These results suggest von Willebrand's syndrome. Her factor VIII level was shown to be reduced at 10%. Von Willebrand's syndrome is an autosomal recessive disorder characterised by mutations within the VIII RAG (von Willebrand's factor, VWF) gene (chromosome 12). This leads to defective function of this protein which has an important role in promoting platelet adhesion to damaged endothelium.

Bleeding episodes in severe von Willebrand's syndrome are treated by infusion of cryoprecipitate, which is rich in VWF, or with intermediate purity factor VIII concentrates, which contain both VWF and factor VIII.

DDAVP (desmopressin) causes increased endogenous production of VWF and is helpful in minor bleeds. Patients must be told to avoid drugs such as aspirin, which can impair platelet function. Screening of family members is advised, and all affected patients should be registered with a haemophilia centre.

Figure **48b** shows cervical lymphadenopathy in a man with Waldenstrom's macroglobulinaemia and an IgM paraprotein, who developed an acquired form of von Willebrand's syndrome in which the paraprotein disturbs interaction between the endothelium and VWF. Bone marrow appearances are shown in **48c**.

48b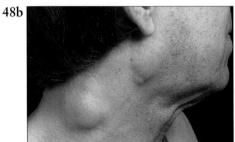

48c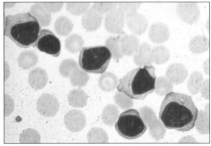

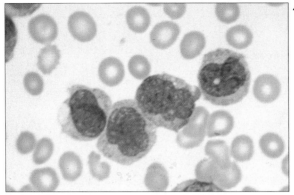

49a

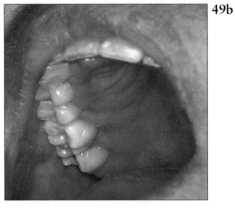

49b

49 i. What abnormality is seen on this blood film (**49a**)?
ii. What abnormality is seen in the patient's mouth (**49b**) and what are the possible causes?
iii. What further investigation would you carry out?

49c

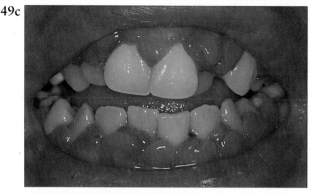

49d

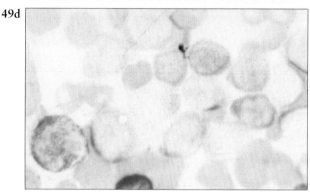

49 i. There are large numbers of atypical blast cells, suggesting a diagnosis of acute leukaemia. These cells have prominent nucleoli, plentiful grey cytoplasm with vacuoles and sparse granules. These features are characteristic of monoblasts, and this is acute monoblastic leukaemia – AML M5.

ii. She has leukaemic infiltration of her gums. M5 AML is often associated with tissue infiltration, and lymphadenopathy, hepatosplenomegaly and nervous system involvement are all commoner than in other types of acute leukaemia. Phenytoin (49c) and cyclosporin therapy are other causes of gum hypertrophy.

iii. She clearly needs bone marrow examination (49d). Monoblasts are usually positive for butyrate esterase (the majority of the cells stain brown on this dual esterase stain; the blue cell is a normal myeloid cell, which is chloroacetate positive). Monoblasts will also stain with the CD14 monoclonal antigen. A serum lysozyme test may be helpful; this is usually raised.

All forms of acute leukaemia, in patients thought suitable for intensive therapy, are treated with combination chemotherapy. Each course typically contains an anthracycline (daunorubicin or idarubicin), cytosine arabinoside and etoposide, and lasts 7–10 days. Supportive care with antibiotics and blood components is critical to success, and most patients have an indwelling central venous (Hickman) catheter.

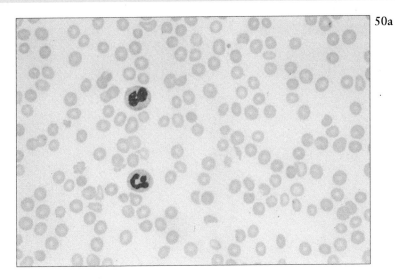

50a

50 A 7-year-old child gives a 7-day history of a brief febrile illness with nausea, vomiting and diarrhoea. Over the past 24 hours, he is noted to have developed purpuric spots over his limbs, and to have become anaemic. Investigations show:

Hb   7 g/dl
WBC   23 x 10⁹/l (neutrophils 83%)
Platelets   11 x 10⁹/l
Urea   49 mmol/l
Creatinine 437 mmol/l
PT   12 seconds (control 11–13 seconds)

i. Comment on the blood film (50a).
ii. What is the likely diagnosis?
iii. What is the pathogenesis of this disorder?
iv. How should the child be treated?

50b

50 i. The blood film shows marked red cell fragmentation, polychromasia and thrombocytopenia.
ii. Haemolytic uraemic syndrome. Henoch–Schönlein purpura is a vasculitis associated with a normal platelet count.
iii. The essential features that define this syndrome are renal microangiopathy, haemolytic anaemia and platelet destruction leading to thrombocytopenia. It is commonest in childhood, and the classic form follows infection with verotoxin-producing strains of *Escherichia coli*, but it is also associated with infections with *Shigella*, *Salmonella* and *Streptococcus*. Bacterial toxins cause endothelial damage, platelet activation, and microangiopathic haemolytic anaemia. Sporadic cases are described in association with auto-immune diseases, pregnancy, the contraceptive pill, radiation nephritis, immune deficiency disorders, and after bone marrow transplantation.
iv. Early and careful management of renal failure and red cell transfusion are the most important aspects of therapy. In adults, this is usually supplemented by fresh frozen plasma therapy or plasma exchange, largely because of the excellent results achieved with this approach in patients with thrombotic thrombocytopenic purpura. Platelet transfusions may have an adverse effect. Isolated reports have supported the use of heparin and anti-platelet drugs. Steroids are not of proven value. Complete recovery is seen in about two-thirds of children, but onset in adulthood usually carries a worse prognosis.

Other causes of red cell fragmentation with haemolysis and thrombocytopenia include disseminated intravascular coagulation (excluded by the normal PT) and microangiopathic haemolytic anaemia (MA HA). which can occur in severe hypertension or in association with disseminated malignancy. Fragmentation haemolysis without thrombocytopenia may occur as a result of mechanical damage to red cells – eg, due to a prosthetic heart valve (50b).

51 A 36-year-old man gives a 3-week history of tiredness, fever and easy bruising. Physical examination shows widespread purpuric lesions. A blood count shows:

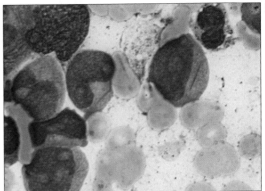
51a

Hb	7.6 g/dl
WBC	33.5 x 10⁹/l
Platelets	5 x 10⁹/l

His bone marrow aspirate is shown (**51a–51c**). He receives 3 courses of intensive chemotherapy followed by allogeneic bone marrow transplantation from a fully histocompatible sibling. 12 days post-transplant he develops weight gain, painful hepatomegaly with jaundice, ascites and renal impairment. He becomes refractory to platelet transfusions.

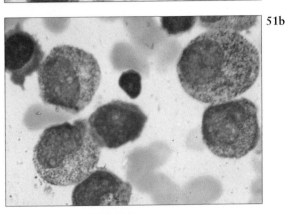
51b

i. What is the presentation diagnosis?
ii. What cytogenetic changes characteristically occur in this disease?
iii. What is the likely cause of his post-transplant complication?

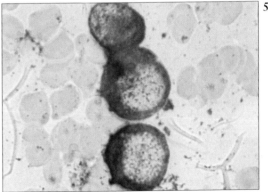
51c

51d

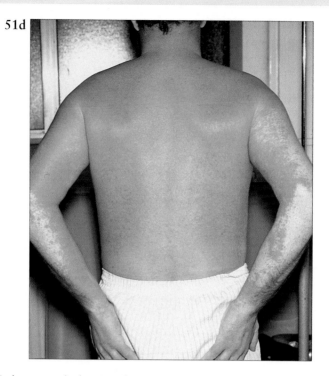

51 i. He has acute leukemia. There is evidence of differentiation of myeloid cells, with granule formation and Auer rods. This is AML M2 in the FAB (French–American–British) classification of acute leukemia.

ii. This patient had translocation t(8:21), which is associated with a good prognosis in AML M2. Other changes in AML include t(15:17) in AML M3 (acute promyelocytic leukaemia), inversion 16 (AML M4 with abnormal eosinophils), trisomy 8 and the Philadelphia chromosome t(9:22) in transformed CGL.

Myelodysplasia is often associated with abnormalities of chromosome 5 and 7; monosomy 7 occurs in AML and in a myelodysplastic/myeloproliferative disorder of infancy.

iii. He has developed veno-occlusive disease. The peak incidence is in the first 2–3 weeks post-allogeneic BMT, and overall incidence is 20–25%. The cause is unknown, but important risk factors are pre-existing liver disease and large doses of previous cytoreductive chemotherapy or high-intensity pre-transplant conditioning. There are ongoing studies evaluating prophylaxis with low dose heparin, pentoxifylline and prostaglandin E1. Treatment is largely supportive but recombinant tissue plasminogen activator has been successfully used to lyse the intrahepatic blood clot.

Acute graft versus host disease (GVHD) also typically presents in the early post-transplant phase. Skin rash (**51d**), often affecting palms and trunk, diarrhoea and abnormal liver function tests occur, but oedema and ascites are uncommon.

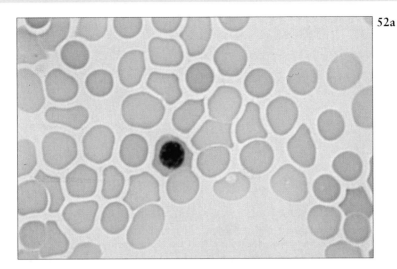

52a

52 A newborn male child is found to be jaundiced and pale at birth. Examination also reveals him to have an easily palpable spleen. The pregnancy was uneventful, even though mother had not attended regularly for antenatal care. She has had one previous uneventful pregnancy. The blood count shows:

Hb   9.5 g/dl
WBC   23.4 x 10⁹/l
Platelets   303 x 10⁹/l

The direct antiglobulin test on cord blood is positive.

i. What abnormalities are seen on this child's blood film (52a)?
ii. What further tests should be performed?
iii. What is the diagnosis?
iv. How is this condition prevented?
v. How is this condition treated?

52b

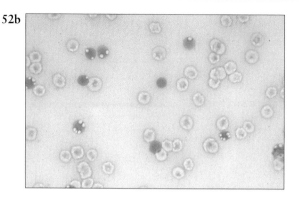

52 i. The blood film shows polychromasia, spherocytes, nucleated red cell and thrombocytopenia, all consistent with an immune haemolytic anaemia. Jaundice at birth is not physiological. The mother's failure to attend for antenatal care means that any atypical red cell antibodies would not have been detected in her serum. Splenomegaly may be normal at birth, but the neonatal Hb should be 16–19 g/dl.

ii. The child's blood group was found to be O Rh(D) positive, while the mother was O Rh(D) negative with a high titre of anti-D antibodies in her serum. The child's DAT is positive, and elution of antibody from child's cells confirmed it to be anti-D. The mother's previous child and the father are both Rh(D) positive, confirming that the mother was sensitised during her previous pregnancy. The child's liver function tests and bilirubin should be assessed, and CMV and rubella infection should be excluded.

iii. Haemolytic disease of fetus and newborn, due to transplacental passage of IgG anti-D from mother to fetus.

iv. Prevention is by administration of anti-D to Rh(D) negative females within 72 hours of a potentially sensitising event, eg, labour, antepartum haemorrhage. The dose of anti-D may need to be increased if the Kleihauer test (52b), which is performed on maternal blood to allow quantification of the number of fetal red blood cells in the maternal circulation, shows a large number present. Fetal haemoglobin can be distinguished from adult haemoglobin by this cytochemical test – the fetal cells stain more darkly.

v. The child may require exchange transfusion with O Rh(D) negative blood, CMV negative, chosen for compatibility with mother's serum. This will lower bilirubin levels (excessive unconjugated bilirubin in fetal blood may damage the neonatal brain – kernicterus). Phototherapy may promote bilirubin conjugation and may be of value.

All pregnant women should be grouped and have a red cell antibody screen performed at booking. If an antibody is detected, its titre should be monitored, and fetal growth closely monitored if the titre is found to be rising. Amniocentesis can be performed after 16–18 weeks' gestation to assess haemolysis. Fetal haemoglobin can be monitored by sampling the umbilical vein under ultrasound guidance. Intrauterine red cell transfusions can be given from about 23–25 weeks' gestation – the blood must be irradiated to prevent graft versus host disease, and it must be from a CMV-negative donor. Plasma exchange can be used to lower the maternal antibody titre.

53 A 19-year-old male presented to his GP with a 3-day history of sore throat. On examination he has an acutely infected throat with bilateral cervical lymphadenopathy. His GP prescribed a course of ampicillin, and the patient developed a widespread erythematous rash (53a). A full blood count shows:

Hb	12.3 g/dl
WBC	7.6 x 10⁹/l (lymphocytes 63%, neutrophils 34%)
Platelets	150 x 10⁹/l

i. Comment on the blood film (53b–53d). What is the diagnosis?
ii. How is the diagnosis confirmed? Indicate the principles involved in the test you describe.
iii. What is the differential diagnosis?
iv. What important complications may occur?

53e

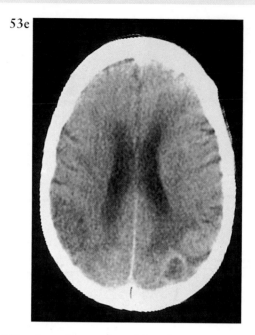

53 **i.** The blood film shows large activated lymphocytes, and there is a relative lymphocytosis in the blood count. The features suggest infectious mononucleosis. A rash following ampicillin therapy is characteristic.
ii. Infectious mononucleosis (glandular fever) is due to infection by the Epstein–Barr virus (EBV), which infects B lymphocytes; the activated lymphocytes seen in the blood film are reactive T lymphocytes. The Paul–Bunnell screening test, or monospot, is a method for detecting a heterophile antibody, which is an antibody that is characteristic of (though not specific for) EBV. This antibody is demonstrated by its failure to be absorbed by guinea pig kidney cells and its ready absorption by ox red blood cells. False-positive results are rare but they can occur, eg, in systemic lupus erythematosus. Detection of antibodies to EBV is a more specific test.
iii. Cytomegalovirus, toxoplasmosis, and adenovirus infections may give a similar blood picture, but they all have a negative monospot.
iv. Generalised lymphadenopathy and splenomegaly are often seen in infectious mononucleosis, and spontaneous rupture of the spleen has been reported. Immune thrombocytopenia, immune haemolytic anaemia, and hepatitis may also occur.
   EBV is implicated in the pathogenesis of nasopharyngeal neoplasia, and it is a co-factor in the development of Burkitt's lymphoma and B cell lymphomas in immunocompromised people, eg, post-transplant patients, HIV-positive patients. Lymphoma in HIV-positive individuals often affects the CNS (53e).

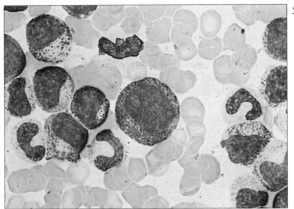

54a

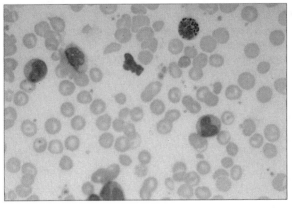

54b

54 A 48-year-old male has noticed a swelling in his left upper abdomen. On examination he has an easily palpable spleen. There is no history of foreign travel, no jaundice, no drug history, and he drinks alcohol in moderation only. There are no signs of chronic liver disease. A full blood count shows:

Hb   14.3 g/dl
WBC   114 x 10⁹/l (neutrophils 84%, blasts 1%, myelocytes 4%,
                    promyelocytes 1%, metamyelocytes 5%, lymphocytes 9%)
Platelets   438 x 10⁹/l

i.   Comment on the blood film (54a, 54b).
ii. What other tests are indicated?
iii. What is the likeliest diagnosis?
iv. How should he be treated?

54 **i.** The blood film shows a neutrophil leukocytosis with immature granulocytic cells present. There are no immature erythroid cells, suggesting that this is a myeloproliferative disorder and not a leukoerythroblastic blood film.

ii. A bone marrow aspirate should be performed and cytogenetic analysis requested. More than 95% of patients with chronic granulocytic (myeloid) leukaemia have a translocation of chromosomal material from 9 to 22 (Philadelphia t9:22 chromosome). This means that the Abelson oncogene is translocated to the breakpoint cluster region (*bcr*) of chromosome 22 and is transcribed to yield a chimeric protein with a tyrosine kinase activity that is many times greater than its normal counterpart. Both aspirate and trephine will show increased cellularity. An abdominal ultrasound is done to confirm splenomegaly.

Baseline liver function tests, urea and electrolytes, and serum LDH should be carried out. A neutrophil alkaline phosphatase (NAP) score (a cytochemical test on fresh peripheral blood neutrophils) will be low (<10, NR 80–120).

iii. Chronic granulocytic leukaemia.

iv. This condition has a fairly benign chronic phase with a median duration of 2.5 years. During this time, patients are well and the disease is easily controlled with oral chemotherapy (eg, hydroxyurea or busulphan).

There is current interest in the use of recombinant interferon, which may prolong this chronic phase of the disease and in a small minority of patients may induce Philadelphia negative haemopoiesis. Bone marrow transplantation is potentially curative during this phase. The disease is usually unresponsive to therapy once transformation (blast crisis) has occurred. Blast crisis may be myeloid or lymphoid in type, but occasionally blast cells will show biphenotypic features. The cells illustated in **54c** showed evidence of both myeloid (CD33, CD13 positive) and lymphoid (CD19 positive, TdT positive) differentiation.

54c

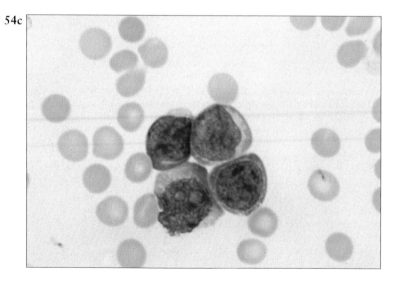

55 A 35-year-old woman has noticed a painless swelling on the left side of her neck, which has been present for over 4 weeks. It is slowly enlarging. There is no relevant past medical history, and no history of fever. Physical examination reveals a single small (1 cm x 0.5 cm) mobile lymph node in the left anterior triangle of the neck. There are no other palpable nodes, and the liver and spleen are not palpable. Investigation shows:

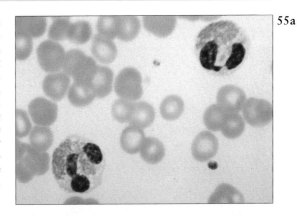
55a

Hb   11.9 g/dl
WBC   8.6 x 10⁹/l
  (neutrophils 5.3 x 10⁹/l,
  eosinophils 1.1 x 10⁹/l,
  lymphocytes 2.1 x 10⁹/l)
Platelets   165 x 10⁹/l

i. Comment on the blood film (55a). What are the important causes of this finding?
ii. Comment on the lymph node biopsy (55b, 55c).
iii. What is the diagnosis?
iv. What further investigations are required?

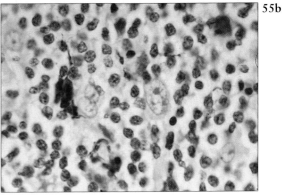
55b

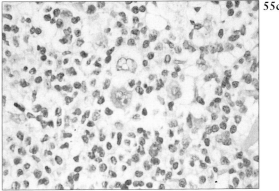
55c

55d 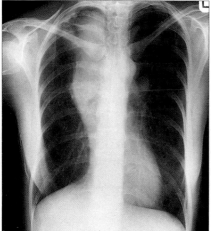 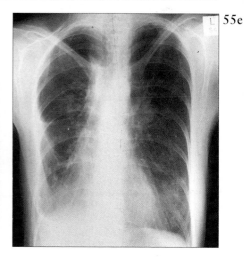 55e

55 i. The film shows increased numbers of eosinophils (NR < 0.4 x 10⁹/l). Important causes of eosinophilia include:

- Allergic reactions (drug hypersensitivity, asthma, eczema).
- Parasitic infections.
- Collagen vascular disease (polyarteritis nodosa).
- Granulomatous conditions (sarcoidosis).
- Neoplasms (haematological neoplasms – eg, lymphoma, acute lymphoblastic leukaemia – and non-haematological neoplasms – eg, breast, bronchus) and idiopathic or primary (eg, hypereosinophilic syndrome).

ii. The lymph node shows a mixed cellular infiltrate with prominent, large Reed–Sternberg cells.
iii. Hodgkin's disease.
iv. Staging, to include a full history (eg, 'B' symptoms would be indicated by pruritus, weight loss and fever), physical examination and investigation.

Investigations would include chest X-ray, thoracic and abdominal CT scans, bone marrow aspirate and trephine biopsy, full haematological and biochemical screen (to include ESR, calcium, immunoglobulins, liver function tests and LDH). A laparotomy is now rarely performed, but it may be valuable in selected cases.

This patient had mediastinal disease (55d) and received treatment with 4 cycles of chemotherapy follwed by radiotherapy ('upper mantle'). Although the chest X-ray taken 2 years later (55e) shows continuing remission from Hodgkin's disease, there is evidence of increased shadowing bilaterally in the lower zones, and she had developed radiation pneumonitis that responded to steroid therapy.

56 A 19-year-old male presents with a 2-week history of bruising and bleeding on brushing his teeth. He has had no serious illness in his past. His girlfriend has noted that over the past few days he has appeared plethoric and his face and eyelids have looked blue, puffy and congested. His full blood count shows:

Hb	9.7 g/dl
WBC	170 x 10⁹/l
Platelets	31 x 10⁹/l

Hb 9.7 g/dl
WBC $170 \times 10^9/l$
Platelets $31 \times 10^9/l$

i. Comment on the chest X-ray (**56a**).
ii. Comment on the blood film (**56b**) and the cytochemistry with acid phosphatase (**56c**). What is the diagnosis? How would you confirm this?
iii. What complications can occur when therapy is commenced, and how would you prevent them?

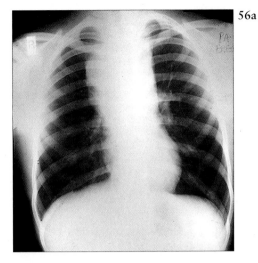

56a

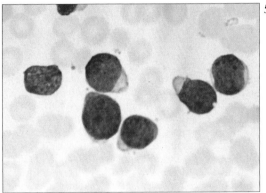

56b

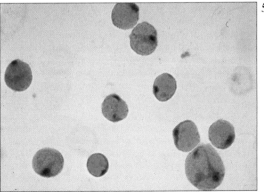

56c

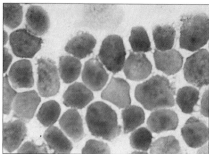

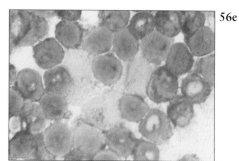

56 i. The chest X-ray shows a mass in the anterior mediastinum, which could be due to lymph nodes or may be thymic in origin. The history suggests he has developed superior vena caval obstruction.

ii. The blood film shows many leukaemic blast cells which are large and have relatively little cytoplasm, prominent nucleoli, and convoluted nuclei. They show positivity for acid phosphatase at their poles ('polar positivity') and are likely to be T cells. The likeliest

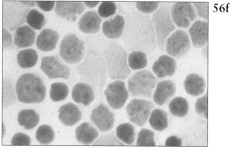

diagnosis is T cell acute lymphoblastic leukaemia, which is often seen in this age group. Confirmation would be by immunocytochemistry with monoclonal antibodies to confirm that the cells are positive for the enzyme TdT (terminal deoxynucleotidyl transferase (56d), and have T cell markers, eg, CD3 (56e). The cells are negative for B cell markers, eg, CD 19 (56f) These monoclonal T cells also have a discrete rearrangement of T cell receptor genes, and this is a specific marker of the disease. It can be used to detect minimal residual disease after chemotherapy.

iii. This is an acute and rapidly proliferating tumour. A tumour lysis syndrome can occur upon commencement of chemotherapy, and disseminated intravascular coagulation may supervene. Metabolic complications include acute renal failure, hypokalaemia, and hypomagnesaemia.

He should be well hydrated with intravenous fluids, and given allopurinol, which blocks the enzyme xanthine oxidase in the liver, and prevents treatment-induced gout and urate nephropathy. Urinary alkalinisation by use of intravenous sodium bicarbonate promotes excretion of harmful metabolites. A good urine output (more than 3 litres daily) should be promoted during therapy.

Initial chemotherapy for acute lymphoblastic leukaemia is with a combination of prednisolone, vincristine, and anthracyclines (eg, daunorubicin), followed by other agents including l-asparaginase and (typically) cytosine arabinoside and etoposide. Maintenance chemotherapy (eg, daily methotrexate and 6-mercaptopurine, and monthly vincristine and prednisolone) should be given for 2 years. Intrathecal and high dose intravenous methotrexate, or possibly craniospinal radiotherapy, are needed to prevent or treat CNS disease.

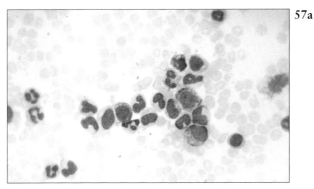

57a

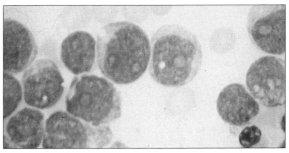

57b

57 A 64-year-old man was noted to have an abnormal blood count at an insurance medical. He was asymptomatic, but on examination had a palpably enlarged spleen . His full blood count showed:

Hb   11.3 g/dl
WBC   73.4 x 10⁹/l
  (blasts 1%, promyelocytes 1%, myelocytes 8%, metamyelocytes 6%,
  neutrophils 76%, lymphocytes 6%, monocytes 2%)
Platelets   430 x 10⁹/l

His NAP score was 8 (NR 60–120), and his liver function tests were normal.
i. What is the likely diagnosis based on the history, the blood count and the blood film(57a)?
ii. He is treated, and remains well for 3 years. A repeat blood count at that time shows:

Hb   8.1 g/dl
WBC   96 x 10⁹/l
Platelets   41 x 10⁹/l

What complication has occurred based on his blood count and blood film (57b) at this time?
iii. What further investigations are warranted?

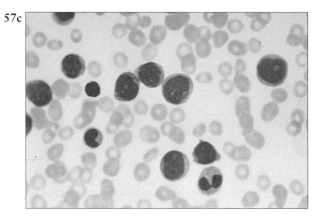

57 i. Chronic granulocytic leukaemia. The blood film shows increased numbers of granulocytic (myeloid) cells at different stages of differentiation. This patient was positive for the Philadelphia chromosome (translocation from 9 to 22). Other forms of chronic myeloid leukaemia include a Philadelphia chromosome negative form, which generally responds less well to therapy; chronic myelomonocytic leukaemia, in which there is a prominent monocytic component, and other forms of myelodysplasia.
ii. The blood film now shows increased numbers of immature blast cells. A bone marrow aspirate would confirm this. Cytochemistry and immunocytochemistry with monoclonal antibodies will help to define the type of leukaemia that has developed. Chronic granulocytic leukaemia usually transforms into a predominantly myeloid form of acute leukaemia (as illustrated here), but often (in approximately 10% of cases) the acute leukaemia is predominantly lymphoid (57c). Although this tends to respond better to therapy, overall prognosis in transformed CGL is very poor, with a median survival of only 16 to 24 weeks. A mixed transformation is often observed.
iii. A repeat cytogenetic investigation is appropriate, as there may be changes additional to the Philadelphia chromosome. Up to 20% of patients are found to have deletion or mutations affecting both alleles of the p53 gene at the time of transformation. p53 is a tumour suppressor gene ('anti-oncogene') and mutations within it are associated with progression of a range of haematological and non-haematological neoplasms. The NAP score usually rises when transformation develops.

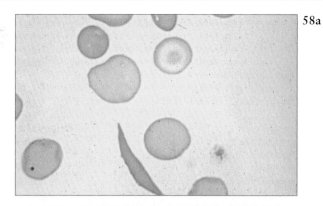

58a

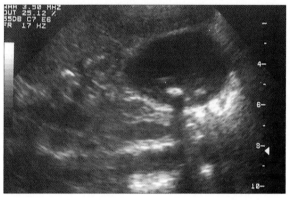

58b

58 An 18-year-old male complains of pain in the right upper abdomen. The pain is colicky and intermittent, and it is associated with fever and jaundice. A blood count shows:

Hb   7.5 g/dl
WBC   27 x 10⁹/l (neutrophils 86%)
Platelets   360 x 10⁹/l

i. What abnormalities are seen on the blood film (58a)?
ii. What is the haematological diagnosis and how would you confirm it?
iii. What abnormality is shown on the abdominal ultrasound scan (58b)?
iv. How should this patient be managed?
v. Six months later he presents with severe tiredness. A blood count shows:

Hb   4.1 g/dl
Reticulocytes 0.1%

What complication has occurred?

58 i. The blood film shows sickle cells, target cells, and Howell–Jolly bodies.
ii. Homozygous sickle cell disease (SS). Auto-infarction of the spleen leads to changes of splenic atrophy in the red blood cells. The polymorph leukocytosis suggests active infection. Confirmation of the diagnosis is by haemoglobin electrophoresis.
iii. The gall bladder contains multiple gallstones.
iv. He should be stabilised with intravenous fluids and antibiotics. If recurrent attacks of cholecystitis occur, cholecystectomy is advised. ERCP may help to exclude biliary obstruction, and it allows contrast studies of the biliary tract to be performed.

Any elective surgery in patients with sickle cell anaemia should be undertaken following exchange transfusion. Thus, at the time of surgery or anaesthesia the level of haemoglobin S should be brought to less than 40% of the total, to minimise the risks of a perioperative sickle cell crisis. Exchange transfusion may also be necessary during pregnancy, and during sickle cell crisis. Red cells for transfusion should be compatible with the patient's own cells for ABO, Kell, and Rh antigens, and for those other red cell antigens which can readily sensitise recipients. The use of hydroxyurea (with or without erythropoietin) and intravenous butyrate therapy to increase haemoglobin F production is under active investigation.
v. Infection with the parvo virus. This leads to 'aplastic crisis' – temporary arrest of erythropoiesis, which is of little consequence to normal individuals, but causes life-threatening anaemia in individuals with hereditary haemolytic anaemia.

The common form of crisis in sickle cell anaemia is due to deoxygenation leading to precipitation of haemoglobin S within red cells, causing shape change and thrombosis. Microvascular occlusion leads to further deoxygenation, and a cycle of sickling is promoted. Precipitating factors are usually not identified, but infection, dehydration and prolonged stasis (eg, following a long aircraft flight) are possible precipitants. Clinical effects may include pain (abdomen, limbs, back), pulmonary sickling (dyspnoea, reduction in arterial oxygen saturation), cerebral sickling (epilepsy, stroke) and priapism. Treatment is with intravenous fluids, analgesia, oxygen and blood transfusion in selected cases.

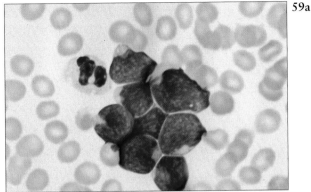
59a

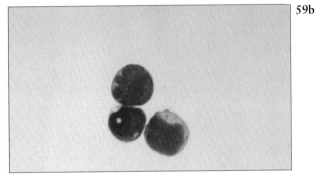
59b

59 A 6-year-old child is assessed in the accident and emergency department, where his parents give a 1-week history of drowsiness, headache, and generalised weakness. His parents concede that he has been generally unwell for 3–4 months, with tiredness and fever. On examination he is pyrexial (38°C) and clearly drowsy, though he responds to verbal commands. He has generalised muscle weakness. There is no neck stiffness. Reflexes are normal and both plantar responses are equivocal. He has generalised lymphadenopathy and liver and spleen are both palpable. A full blood count shows:

Hb	$7.6 \times 10^9/l$
WBC	$137 \times 10^9/l$
Platelets	$34 \times 10^9/l$

i. Comment on the blood film appearances (**59a**).
ii. A lumbar puncture is performed. Comment on the appearances of the cells in the cerebrospinal fluid (**59b**).
iii. What is the diagnosis and how would you confirm it?
iv. What other tissues may be involved by this condition?

59c

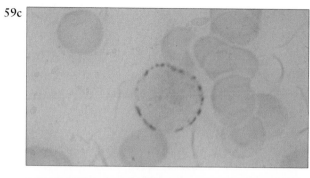

59d

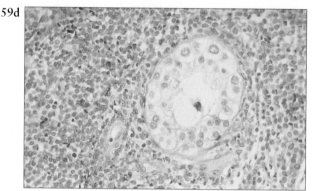

59 i. The blood film shows large numbers of primitive cells, with scanty cytoplasm, no granules and positivity for PAS (Periodic Acid Schiff reaction, **59c**) with blocks of positive material.

ii. Cells similar to the peripheral blood are seen on this cytospin preparation of cerebrospinal fluid.

iii. Acute lymphoblastic leukaemia (ALL) with central nervous system (CNS) involvement. The PAS reaction is important confirmatory evidence, but the cells were also positive by immunocytochemistry for the CD10 (common ALL) antigen. They were B cells (CD19 positive), and had a discrete rearrangement of their immunoglobulin heavy-chain genes.

iv. Testicular (**59d**) and ovarian disease are well recognised. All children with ALL are at risk of CNS disease, and treatment aimed at preventing CNS disease should be offered in presymptomatic patients. Such treatment includes intrathecal chemotherapy, high-dose treatment with chemotherapeutic drugs that cross the blood–brain barrier (eg, methotrexate, cytosine arabinoside), and possibly craniospinal radiotherapy.

The overall prognosis for childhood ALL is very good, and more than 60% of patients are cured. Children who do less well include those with a high presenting white cell count (>50 x 10⁹/l), boys, children aged under 2 or over 12 years, and those with CNS disease at presentation. Normal cytogenetics and hyperdiploidy indicate good prognosis; the Philadelphia translocation (t[9;22]), t(4;11) and t(1;19) indicate poor prognosis.

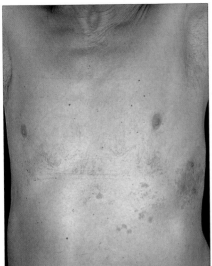

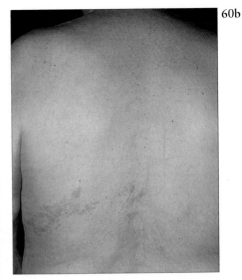

60 A 76-year-old man presented with an intensely painful and itchy rash across his lower chest. A full blood count shows:

Hb   12.1 g/dl
WBC   76 x 10⁹/l
 (lymphocytes 91%, neutrophils 8%)
Platelets   117 x 10⁹/l
Examination also revealed generalised

lymphadenopathy and a palpable spleen.
i. What is the dermatological diagnosis (60a, 60b), and how should he be treated?
ii. What abnormality is shown on the blood film (60c), and what is the haematological diagnosis?
iii. What basic therapies are available for his blood condition?
iv. What variants of this haematological condition are recognised?

60: Answers

60d
60e 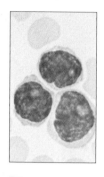 60f

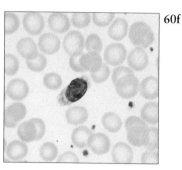 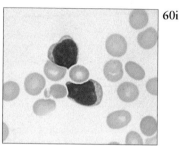

60g
60h 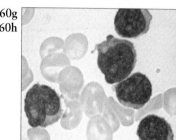 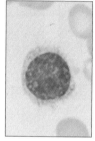 60i

60 i. The rash is typical of shingles (herpes zoster). This condition should be treated with high doses of acyclovir, preferably intravenously.

ii. The blood film shows increased numbers of mature lymphoid cells and increased numbers of damaged, or smear, cells. Similar cells are seen in the marrow (**60d**). These findings suggest chronic lymphocytic leukaemia.

iii. These patients are at increased risk of infection (because of hypogammaglobuli-naemia), and they may need supportive care and treatment of complications such as immune haemolytic anaemia and immune thrombocytopenia. Many patients need no therapy at all, and stable disease should be observed and monitored. Progressive disease is treated initially with single agent chemotherapy (eg, chlorambucil), but patients with bulky or progressive disease and bone marrow failure may need combination therapy. Newer agents, such as fludarabine and 2-chlorodeoxyadenosine, are being evaluated. Splenectomy and radiotherapy to bulky lymph nodes are other forms of therapy.

iv. Variants of chronic lymphocytic leukaemia include:
- B cell CLL (as in this patient) carries a good prognosis (10 or more years).
- T cell CLL (**60e**) is rare, responds less well to therapy, and often affects the skin.
- Splenic lymphoma with villous lymphocytes (SLVL) (**60f**), which is often accompanied by a paraprotein and responds well to splenectomy.
- B cell prolymphocytic leukaemia is characterised by larger cells with nucleoli (**60g**) may evolve in patients with CLL or may appear *de novo*. The white cell count is usually markedly raised, splenomegaly is common, and response to therapy is often poor.
- Hairy cell leukaemia (**60h**) is usually B cell but occasionally T cell type.
- Follicular lymphoma (**60i**) affecting the peripheral blood, which can give rise to a similar appearance.

124

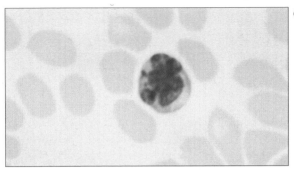

61a

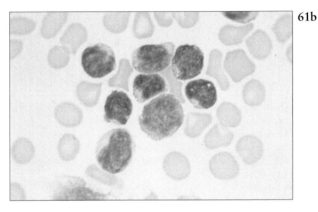

61b

61 A 40-year-old West Indian has bilateral axillary lymphadenopathy. He has a 3- to 4-week history of gradually increasing weakness and stiffness of both legs, with lack of sensation. His full blood count shows:

Hb	11.1 g/dl
WBC	39 x 10⁹/l
Platelets	91 x 10⁹/l

Biochemical analysis shows:

Urea	13 mmol/l
Na⁺	142 mmol/l
K⁺	5.5 mmol/l
Ca²⁺	3.15 mmol/l
Albumin	38 g/l
Alkaline phosphatase 1	35 IU/l

i. Comment on the blood film (**61a, 61b**).
ii. What further tests would you do?
iii. What is the diagnosis, treatment and prognosis?

61c

61 i. The film shows atypical lymphocytes with convoluted nuclei. He has hypercalcaemia and a history compatible with transverse myelitis.
ii. The following tests should be carried out:

• Serology for HTLV1 (human T cell lymphoma virus), a retroviral infection that is endemic in the Caribbean and Japan.
• A lymph node biopsy.
• Staging investigations, which should include chest and abdominal CT scans, bone marrow and serum LDH.
• Immunophenotype analysis of peripheral-blood T cells to confirm they are T cells.

iii. Acute T cell leukaemia/lymphoma. This is a high-grade lymphoma, best treated with aggressive combination chemotherapy.
   This patient also requires hydration and steroid or biphosphonate therapy for his hypercalcaemia. This tumour is typically very aggressive and responds poorly to therapy. They are positive for the T cell antigens CD2, CD3 (**61c**) and CD5, and usually CD4 (helper T cell) positive and CD8 (suppressor T cell) negative.

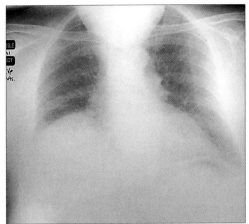

62a

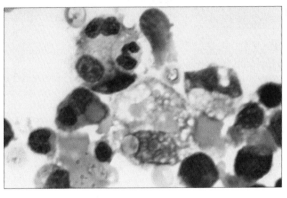

62b

62 A 35-year-old patient has a 4- to 6-week history of fever, loss of weight, anorexia and malaise. He has no fixed abode, and also complains of an irritating cough with purulent sputum. Examination shows him to be unkempt and pyrexial (his temperature is 39°C). He has cervical lymphadenopathy. He also has bruises over his legs. Investigations show:

Hb	6.5 g/dl
MCV	84 fl
WBC	$2.9 \times 10^9/l$
Platelets	$34 \times 10^9/l$

i. Comment on the chest X-ray findings (**62a**).
ii. Comment on the bone marrow aspirate (**62b**).
iii. What is the haematological diagnosis and what conditions may be associated with it?
iv. What further tests should be done?

62c

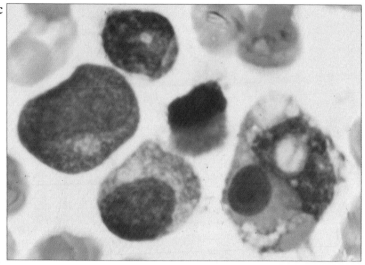

62 i. There are bilateral changes of widespread reticulonodular shadowing which, with this history, would be consistent with miliary tuberculosis.
ii. There are abnormal macrophages which have engulfed mature red cells, white cells, and platelets. The changes suggest haemophagocytic syndrome (see also **62c**).
iii. This may occur in association with infection (eg, tuberculosis or viral infections) particularly in immunosuppressed patients. It may be associated with neoplasia (eg, malignant lymphoma) or be part of a primary histocytic neoplasm (eg, histocytic medullary reticulosis). It is also reported in association with auto-immune conditions.
iv. An HIV test should be performed.

63 A 65-year-old man developed back pain over a 4-week period. He was otherwise well. Investigations showed:

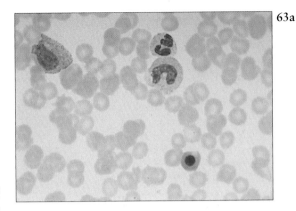

63a

Hb   9.1 g/dl
WBC   12.7 x 10⁹/l
(neutrophils 62%, lymphocytes 31%, metamyelocytes 2%, myelocytes 1%, monocytes 2%, eosinophils 1%, basophils 1%)
Platelets   137 x 10⁹/l
NRBC:WBC   1:100 (ratio of nucleated red blood cells to white cells)
ESR   82 mm/hour

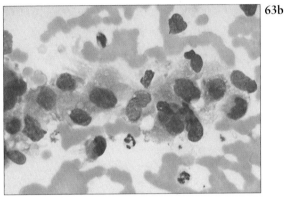

63b

i. Comment on the differential white cell count and blood film (**63a**).
ii. Comment on the bone marrow aspirates (**63b** and **63c**).
iii. What further tests are indicated?
iv. The patient underwent a retropubic prostatectomy, but postoperatively he developed severe haematuria which persisted for 12 hours despite bladder washouts.
Tests showed:

Hb   6.1 g/dl
Platelets   131 x 10⁹/l
PT   15 seconds
(control 11–13 seconds)
APTT   45 seconds
(control 30–40 seconds)
APTT mix with normal plasma 50:50   35 seconds
Thrombin time 40 seconds
(control 15–20 seconds)
Fibrinogen   0.01
(NR 2.0–4.0 g/l)
Fibrin degradation products
(FDP)   >1:160
(NR <1:10)

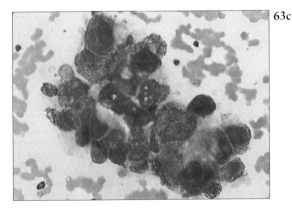

63c

What complication has occurred, and how should he be treated?

63d

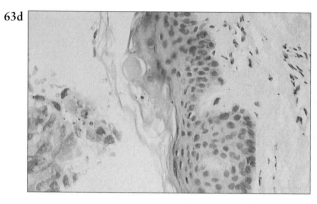

63e

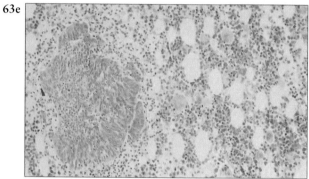

63 i. He has a leukoerythroblastic blood film, which suggests marrow infiltration by abnormal non-myeloid cells. This is an indication for marrow examination.

ii. The aspirate and trephine biopsy show infiltration by abnormal cells – glandular elements are clearly visible in the trephine biopsy. The appearances suggest secondary carcinoma. He also has back pain. Also shown are cells from a carcinoma of the stomach in a bone marrow trephine (63d), and a trephine biopsy of oat cell carcinoma of the bronchus (63e).

iii. The prostatic specific antigen was raised. The cells in the aspirate were positive for acid phosphatase, and a bone scan also showed secondary deposits. Rectal examination and prostatic biopsy confirmed the diagnosis.

iv. His haemoglobin has dropped and he needs blood component therapy. Disseminated intravascular coagulation is a possibility, but the platelet count is normal. The prolonged thrombin time, the profoundly lowered fibrinogen level and the raised FDP after the prostatic surgery suggest hyperfibrinolysis. The prostate bed is a rich source of plasminogen activators which cause fibrin degradations; D–D dimers (formed also from fibrin degradation) would be raised.

He should have therapy with tranexamic acid or EACA, both of which are specific inhibitors of plasminogen activators.

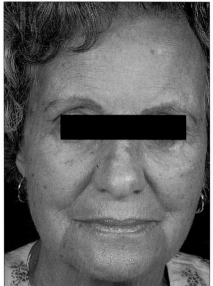

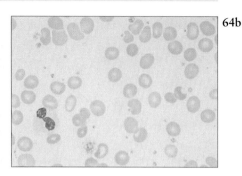

64 An 82-year-old woman has been treated for 5 months for persisting anaemia and thrombocytopenia. Her full blood count shows:

Hb   7.1 g/dl
WBC   1.3 x 10⁹/l (neutrophils 40%, lymphocytes 45%, blasts 2%)
Platelets   23 x 10⁹/l

i.   Comment on the appearance of this patient's face (**64a**).
ii. Comment on the appearance of the blood film (**64b**).
iii. What is the diagnosis?
iv. What is the prognosis of this condition?

64: Answers

64c
64d

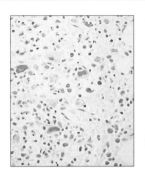

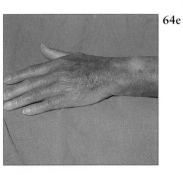

64e

64f

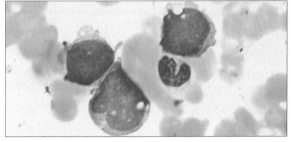

64 i. The face shows a greyish pigmentation which is due to transfusional iron overload. The bone marrow aspirate (Perl's stain) shows increased iron (64c), and the trephine biopsy shows increased haemosiderin (64d). Other complications of the iron overload include endocrinopathy (eg, diabetes), liver disease, and cardiomyopathy. This patient also had extensive ecchymosis (64e) as a result of her thrombocytopenia.
ii. The blood film shows hyposegmentation of neutrophil nuclei (pseudo-Pelger forms) with hypogranularity, an occasional blast, and platelet/red cell anisocytosis.
iii. Myelodysplasia. This is characterised by cytopenias affecting more than one lineage in the face of a cellular marrow, indicating defective maturation within the marrow. Abnormal megakaryocytes and blasts are other typical features in myelodysplasia (64f).
iv. Myelodysplasia typically affects elderly people (but can occur at any age) and is a disorder of the haemopoietic stem cell. Cytogenetic changes are frequently seen, and these most commonly affect chromosomes 5 and 7. Genetic mutations affecting growth and differentiation of haemopoietic stem cells are involved in the pathogenesis of these preleukaemic disorders, but the precise cause is not known. Some patients have previously had myelosuppressive chemotherapy for an unrelated neoplasm.

Prognosis depends on the degree of cytopenia (which influences the risk of complications of bone marrow failure) and the proportion of blasts in blood and bone marrow (which influences the risk of leukaemic transformation). Patients with early myelodysplasia (eg, refractory anaemia with or without ringed sideroblasts) may need no therapy and have a median survival of 4–6 years. Patients with chronic myelomonocytic leukaemia and refractory anaemia with excess blasts (RAEB) have a median survival of approximately 1 year, whereas patients with more than 20% of bone marrow blasts (RAEB in transformation) or 30% blasts (AML) should receive AML therapy if they are considered able to tolerate intensive therapy.

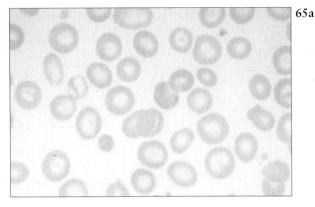

65a

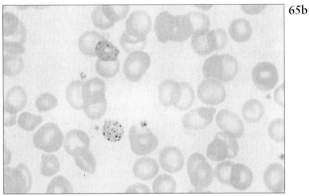

65b

65 A 40-year-old Indian man is referred for investigation of anaemia. He has also complained recently of abdominal pain with nausea. He has had no serious illnesses in the past, and his only medications are herbal remedies. A full blood count shows:

Hb	8.2 g/dl
MCV	95 fl
WBC	normal
Platelets	normal

i. What abnormality is seen on the blood film (65a, 65b)?
ii. What is the diagnosis?
iii. What further investigations/treatment would you recommend?

65c

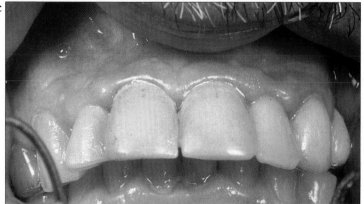

65 i. Basophilic stippling within the red cells.
ii. Lead poisoning, which is presumably related to a herbal remedy.
iii. The herbal preparation should be sent for analysis, and other users and the manufacturers should be alerted. A serum lead level should be performed.

Lead poisoning may also explain the abdominal pain, and it can cause encephalopathy, circulatory collapse and muscle cramps. Lead interferes with the haem biosynthetic pathway, and the level of urinary delta amino laevulinic acid is elevated. Treatment in acute stages of lead poisoning, if excessive ingestion is recent and particularly if there is encephalopathy, should include gastric lavage and instillation of a chelating agent in the stomach, eg, d-penicillamine. Oral d-penicillamine can be repeated 3 times daily and is particularly suitable in children.

Other causes of basophilic stippling include thalassaemia, myelodysplasia, immune haemolytic anaemia, alcohol, and congenital enzymopathies (eg, pyrimidine-5'-nucleotidase deficiency), megaloblastic anaemia and sideroblastic anaemia.

Figure 65c shows his teeth and gums, and the characteristic blue lead line in his gums.

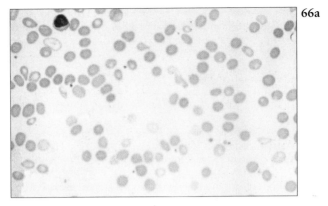

66a

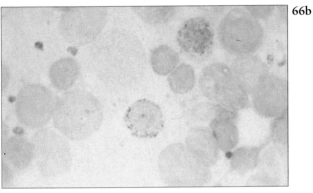

66b

66 **i.** What abnormality is shown in this blood film (66a)?
ii. What are the possible causes?
iii. What abnormality is shown in the bone marrow aspirate (66b)?
iv. What is the treatment?

66 i. The blood film shows a dimorphic population of red blood cells, and is from a patient with sideroblastic anaemia. One population of red cells is hypochromic while the other has a normal haemoglobin content. Other causes of 2 red cell populations include:

• Mixed iron and B_{12}–folate deficiency.
• Acute haemorrhage.
• Blood transfusion.

ii. Sideroblastic anaemia is characterised by defective synthesis of haem. This can be caused by an inherited condition (which is rare, and is typically seen as a sex-linked recessive). It is more commonly an acquired condition; causes include:

• Myelodysplasia (refractory anaemia with ringed sideroblasts, RARS, probably the same condition as primary or idiopathic acquired sideroblastic anaemia).
• Drugs (alcohol, chloramphenicol, isoniazid).
• Lead poisoning.
• Vitamin B_6 (pyridoxine) deficiency.

(Note that RARS, as part of myelodysplasia, is often associated with thrombocytopenia or leukopenia, and is a clonal, pre-leukaemic condition.)
iii. The iron (Perl's) stain shows ringed sideroblasts – abnormal accumulation of iron granules within the mitochondria and distributed in a circular fashion around the nucleus.
iv. Treatment depends on the cause, and persistent symptomatic anaemia usually requires blood transfusion.

Vitamin B_6 is the co-factor for the enzyme delta-amino-laevulinic acid synthetase, which is an important step in haem synthesis. Isoniazid therapy should be combined with vitamin B_6 supplements to prevent sideroblastic anaemia.

67 A 76-year-old man has a 2- to 3-week history of headache and lethargy. He smokes 15 cigarettes daily but does not have a history of chronic lung disease. His appetite is good and his weight is steady. He has also noticed generalised pruritus after a shower.

Examination reveals a palpable spleen. Investigations show:

Hb	19.6 g/dl
MCV	76 fl
RBC	7.4 x 10⁹/l
PCV	0.59 fl
WBC	16.1 x 10⁹/l
(neutrophils 66%)	
Platelets	452 x 10⁹/l

Hb 19.6 g/dl
MCV 76 fl
RBC $7.4 \times 10^9/l$
PCV 0.59 fl
WBC $16.1 \times 10^9/l$
(neutrophils 66%)
Platelets $452 \times 10^9/l$

i. Comment on this patient's facial appearance (**67a**).

ii. What are the causes of a raised haemoglobin?

iii. What further tests are indicated?

iv. What is the diagnosis?

v. How should he be treated?

The patient subsequently went on to develop a generalised, intensely pruritic skin rash over his trunk (**67b**), associated with abdominal pain and diarrhoea. A repeat bone marrow examination (**67c**) was carried out at this stage.

vi. What condition has now developed?

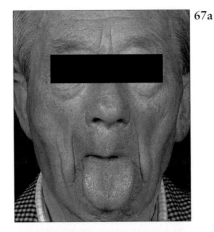

67a

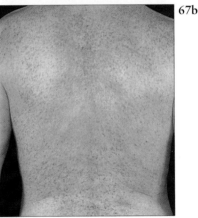

67b

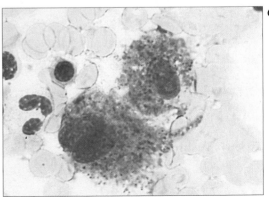

67c

67 i. He has plethora.
ii. A raised haemoglobin may
be due to a true erythrocytosis
(or polycythaemia) or it may
be spurious (or relative).
Spurious polycythaemia
occurs as a concentration effect
in people with reduced plasma
volume ('stress polycythaemia').
This is seen in hypertension,
during diuretic therapy, and in
association with smoking.
True polycythaemia may be
appropriate (or physiological),
eg, at high altitude, in people
with chronic lung disease or

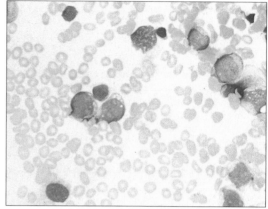

67d

cyanotic congenital heart disease, or in association with a high oxygen affinity
haemoglobin variant. Inappropriate polycythaemia occurs in response to an erythro-
poietin-secreting tumour (eg, renal cysts, hypernephroma, uterine and hepatic
tumours) or in primary proliferative polycythaemia (PPP), which is a myeloproliferative disorder.

iii. The presence of splenomegaly strongly suggests PPP, but an abdominal ultrasound
should be performed to confirm that the abdominal mass is not an enlarged kidney.

A urate level should be documented, as these patients are at increased risk of
developing gout. The neutrophil alkaline phosphatase score is usually raised in PPP.

Pulmonary function tests will exclude long-standing lung disease as a contributory
cause for the raised haemoglobin.

More than 50% of patients with PPP have raised white cell and platelet counts as
part of their myeloproliferative disorder. A red cell mass and plasma volume estimation is useful to document the presence of a true polycythaemia.

iv. Polycythaemia rubra vera, or primary proliferative polycythaemia.

v. The aim in PPP is to maintain the PCV at less than 0.45, as this reduces the risk of
thrombosis. This is most easily achieved with regular venesection, but chemotherapy
(eg, oral hydroxyurea, busulphan or intermittent 32P) may be required. Iron therapy
should be avoided.

Patients with myeloproliferative disorder have an increased risk of developing
leukaemia, and some therapies (eg, chlorambucil and other alkylating agents, and
32P) have been shown to increase the risk further. A bone marrow aspirate is shown
(67d) from a patient with PPP, treated with long-term 32P, who has developed acute
myelomonocytic leukaemia.

Low-dose antiplatelet therapy (eg, aspirin 150 mg on alternate days) will reduce
the thrombotic tendency.

vi. The bone marrow shows infiltration by mast cells. This, together with the skin
rash, suggests he has developed systemic mastocytosis, which is associated with the
myeloproliferative disorders.

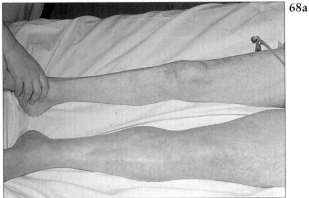

68a

68 A 28-year-old male presents with a 1-week history of gradually increasing pain and swelling of his left leg (68a). Over the previous 24 hours he has coughed up blood-stained sputum on 2 occasions. His father died suddenly of unknown causes at the age of 46 and his 27-year-old sister suffered a deep vein thrombosis during pregnancy.
Investigations show:

Hb   13.4 g/dl
WBC   7.9 x 10⁹/l
Platelets   313 x 10⁹/l
PT   12 seconds (control 11–13 seconds)
APTT   34 seconds (control 30–40 seconds)

i. What is the diagnosis and how would you confirm it?
ii. What additional investigations should be performed?
iii. What therapeutic options should be considered?

68b

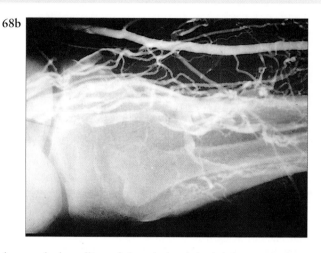

68 **i.** He has marked swelling of the whole of the left leg suggesting an ileofemoral venous thrombosis. A venogram should be performed to confirm this; the illustration (**68b**) shows the presence of thrombus in the deep veins of the calf and popliteal region. The history of haemoptysis suggests a pulmonary embolism (which may also have been the cause of his father's death). This may be confirmed by a ventilation/perfusion isotope scan but pulmonary angiography should be considered as he may be a candidate for surgery.

ii. He should be screened for the presence of a familial hypercoagulable state due to deficiency of one of the inhibitors of coagulation, e.g. anti-thrombin III, protein C and protein S. These are autosomal dominant disorders associated with an increased risk of both venous and arterial thrombosis, often presenting at a young age. The diagnosis in this case was anti-thrombin III deficiency, which is a heterogeneous disorder in which many molecular variants of anti-thrombin III are recognised. Protein C inactivates Factors V and VIII; resistance to activated protein C is one of the commonest causes of inherited 'thrombophilia', and can arise as a result of a single mutation in the Factor V gene. Rarer inherited causes include defects of fibrinogen or of plasminogen activators. Acquired disorders which lead to hypercoagulability include the presence of the lupus anticoagulant in SLE, paroxysmal nocturnal haemoglobinuria and thrombocytosis.

iii. He requires treatment with thrombolytic therapy, provided there are no contraindications (eg, recent surgery or active peptic ulceration). Streptokinase and urokinase are given as a loading dose followed by maintenance therapy monitored by clinical and laboratory (prolongation of thrombin time) response. Newer plasminogen activators – eg, tissue plasminogen activator – may be safer by activating plasminogen locally rather than systemically. They are under evaluation.

Other therapeutic options include:
• Insertion of a filter device (eg, Greenfield filter) in the inferior vena cava.
• Surgical thrombectomy: this should be considered for the pulmonary embolism.
• Anticoagulation with heparin followed by oral warfarin: while this may prevent clot propagation it will not lyse thrombus.

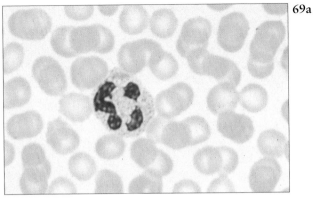

69a

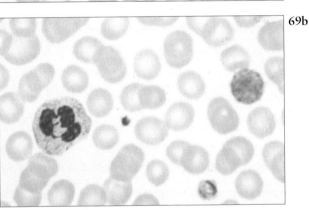

69b

69 A 50-year-old woman has excessive bleeding following tooth extraction. She has never had excessive bleeding before, and there is no relevant family history. She has had two normal vaginal deliveries in the past. Physical examination is normal. Investigations show:

Hb	13.5 g/dl
WBC	6.7 x 10⁹/l
Platelets	80 x 10⁹/l
PT	12 seconds (control 11–13 seconds)
APTT	39 seconds (control 30–40 seconds)
Ivy template bleeding time	4 minutes (normal range up to 10 minutes)

i. Comment on her blood film appearances (69a and 69b) and on the above results.
ii. Discuss the differential diagnosis.

69c

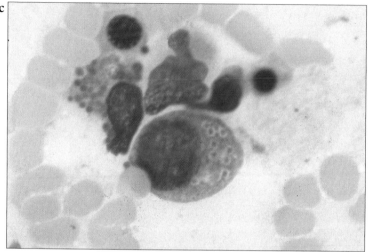

69 i. The blood film shows giant platelets. The neutrophil has an abnormal inclusion which is similar to the Dohle body, found as a feature of neutrophils responding to severe infection. There is a mild thrombocytopenia. The clinical history suggests she may have a mild bleeding disorder, but the coagulation tests and bleeding time are normal.

ii. This patient suffers from the May–Hegglin anomaly, a rare, dominantly inherited disorder which runs a benign course. Bleeding manifestations are rare and platelet function studies are essentially normal. Bernard–Soulier syndrome is an autosomal recessive or codominant trait also associated with giant platelets and thrombocytopenia; but there are no neutrophil inclusions, bleeding manifestations are common and platelet membranes lack glycoprotein 1b and fail to aggregate in response to ristocetin.

Giant platelets may be confused with red cells by automatic cell counters to lead to a spurious thrombocytopenia. They also occur in myelodysplasia, myelofibrosis and as part of thrombocytosis in essential thrombocythaemia and iron deficiency. Giant platelets with thrombocytopenia appear as a benign abnormality in certain Mediterranean populations and is reported in Down's syndrome and with autosomal dominant nephritis and deafness (Epstein's syndrome).

Chediak–Higashi syndrome (**69c**) is a rare autosomal recessive condition wherein partial ocular and cutaneous albinism are associated with a bleeding tendency, severe granulocyte functional abnormalities and abnormal inclusions in developing and mature myeloid cells.

70a 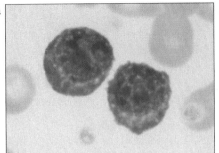 70b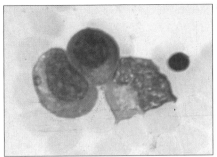

70 A 58-year-old female gives a 4-week history of being generally unwell. She has had intermittent fever, loss of appetite and has lost almost 4 kilos (8 pounds) in weight over 2 months. She has had joint pains affecting hands, wrists and ankles which have persisted despite treatment with diclofenac. She developed a generalised skin rash 3 days after commencing a course of amoxycillin. Some 6 months previously she had developed hypothyroidism.

Examination reveals a pale lady who appears ill. She has generalised lymphadenopathy in the cervical, axillary and inguinal regions, and both liver and spleen are palpable. She has swelling of the proximal interphalangeal joints and wrists and a faint macular rash affecting her trunk and upper part of her thighs. Investigation shows:

Hb	8.6 g/dl
MCV	81 fl
WBC	11.6 x 10⁹/l
Platelets	65 x 10⁹/l
Urea	9.8 mmol/l
AST	320 (normal 5–40 units/l)
ALT	170 (normal 5–40 units/l)
Alkaline phosphatase	275 (normal 35–130 units/l)
ESR	110 mm/hour

Protein electrophoresis shows a faint paraprotein band (later characterised as IgG kappa, 6 g/l) with remaining immunoglobulins at the lower limit of normal.
A bone marrow aspirate is performed.

i. Comment on the appearances of the blood film (70a) and bone marrow (70b).
ii. What is the differential diagnosis?
iii. What further management would you suggest?

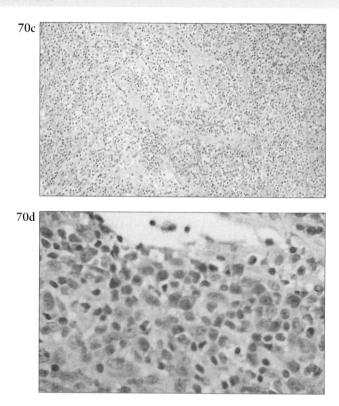

70c

70d

70 i. The peripheral blood film (70a) shows circulating differentiated B lymphocytes that are plasma cells. Figure 70b shows similar cells (plasma cells or immunoblasts) in the marrow.

ii. The clinical history, with skin rash, arthralgia, drug sensitivity, lymphadenopathy, fever, organomegaly and past history of endocrinopathy, is classical for angioimmunoblastic lymphadenopathy with dysproteinaemia (AILD). Auto-immune thrombocytopenia and haemolytic anaemia frequently occur. Lymph node biopsy (70c) characteristically shows effacement of architecture with arborisation of blood vessels (the angio-component of AILD) and a higher power view of the node (70d) shows a polymorphous infiltrate with numerous immunoblasts. A high proportion of patients have clonal rearrangements of T cell receptor and/or immunoglobulin genes and the condition progresses to overt lymphoma in about a third of cases. Differential diagnosis is wide and includes connective tissue disease, drug hypersensitivity, infection (eg, viral hepatitis, bacterial endocarditis), lymphoma and myeloma.

iii. Further diagnostic procedures (eg, lymph node biopsy, liver biopsy if coagulation tests permit, CT scan, autoimmune serology, and urine examination for paraprotein, protein and casts) are required. Lymph node biopsy was diagnostic in this case. Therapeutic options for AILD are wide and include immunosuppressive therapy (eg, steroids, cyclophosphamide) and intensive combination chemotherapy with a lymphoma regime. Prognosis is poor and 2 year survival is only 30%.

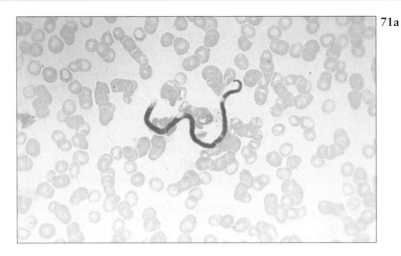
71a

71 i. What abnormality is seen on this blood film (71a)?
ii. What haematological changes commonly accompany this abnormality?
iii. How is this condition treated?

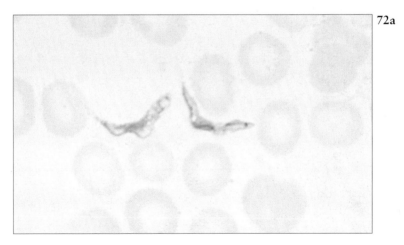
72a

72 A 27-year-old male has recently returned from southern Africa. He complains of intermittent fever. His full blood count shows:

Hb   7.1 g/dl
WBC   17.5 x 10^9/l (eosinophils 4 x 10^9/l, lymphocytes 9 x 10^9/l)
Platelets   56 x 10^9/l

i. What is the diagnosis (72a)?
ii. What other haematological complications may occur?

145

71 i. Filariasis, probably due to *Wuchereria bancrofti*. The larvae are transmitted by mosquito bites, adult worms then develop in the lymphatics, and mature females release microfilariae into the blood stream. These microfilariae are ingested by biting mosquitoes.

ii. Eosinophilia (1–30 x 10^9/l) and lymphocytosis are frequently seen. Tropical eosinophilia is associated with dyspepsia, wheezing, chest pain and pyrexia, and is frequently due to occult filariasis with pulmonary and lymphatic involvement.

iii. Treatment is with oral diethylcarbamazine which is usually given for 21 days.

72 i. Trypanosomiasis, probably due to *Trypanosoma rhodesiense*.

ii. Splenomegaly is frequently seen. Anaemia is due to haemolysis, caused by release of haemolysins by trypanosomes, erythrophagocytosis within the reticuloendothelial system and splenomegaly with pooling. Thrombocytopenia arises through splenic pooling and DIC.

Index

148